DEBORAH A. NEWKIRK
YOUTH VOLLEYBALL
CURRICULUM

Presented by

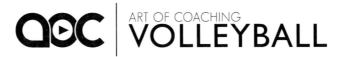

Printed in the United States of America

First Printing, 2017

ISBN 978-0-9989765-4-9

Published by The Art of Coaching Volleyball, LLC

3720 SW 141st Avenue, Suite 209
Beaverton, OR 97005

www.theartofcoachingvolleyball.com

Table of Contents

Foreword from Deborah Newkirk

Hi there! Deborah Newkirk here. With over three decades of experience in youth coaching, I'm a physical educator who has spent a professional lifetime bringing the worlds of coaching and teaching together. After twenty years of competitive coaching, I began focusing on training and created COACH 'EM UP. Today, COACH 'EM UP serves as a resource for nearly 3,000 families a year. Year round off-the-floor training programs have been a big part of the COACH 'EM UP success, providing young athletes with motivation and an organized means of improving their game, both on the court and in their backyards.

My story started with me landing a job that threw me into a coaching position in a sport where I had very little experience and know-how. Volleyball was not my number one sport. In my mind, there was only one thing to do in this situation - seek out knowledge and become the strongest teacher possible.

As a young professional, I couldn't gather books quickly enough from The Greats! Attending every clinic, scheduling meetings to learn from other coaches, going to college practices and matches, making phone calls to discuss the difference between the 5-1 and 6-2 offense, understanding rotations and how to "get all my kids in" the match has made me a true student of the game. Three things that I learned early on still hold true today (three decades later): to be professionally prepared, set goals for short-term progress and long-time learning; to teach with confidence in your subject matter; and to deliver your message with a language that connects with your audience whether they are a big-time talented team or a room full of eager first graders.

As a physical educator, I have loved writing the curriculum. Professionally speaking, it may be one of the greatest joys I've experienced in teaching. The Youth Volleyball Curriculum is about a system. It offers an educator one lesson that feeds into the next to create a seamless introduction of skill sets with a series of matching muscle-memory based touches. It blends fun challenges on the court with age-appropriate homework that reinforces progress. With skills comes confidence, and with confidences comes... well, whatever they aspire to do and be. The games, drills, and skill progressions have years behind them, and many, many players have endorsed the product - if you consider smiling faces and a strong base of fundamentals an endorsement!

Enjoy and thank you!

Deborah A. Newkirk

How it Works

The Youth Volleyball Curriculum is designed to be used by youth coaches, PE teachers, volunteer coaches, and gym or sport directors working with players ranging from ages 5 to 12.

The curriculum was developed to prepare the instructor with a plan that includes a library of cue words, phrases and drills to reinforce their instruction of the game of volleyball.

Use the book in three easy steps:
1. Identify the age or skill level of the group you are working with
2. Prepare your daily or weekly practice plan by following the week-by-week schedule for that level
3. Use the lessons, drills, challenges, etc. listed under that week's schedule to teach and expand your players' volleyball knowledge.

How to use the different sections of the book:
- **Drill Key:** Teaches you what each symbol represents in the drill diagrams throughout the book.
- **Year Introduction:** Each year of instruction includes an introduction that explains what to expect from the players of that level and what skills suit their age best.
- **Practice Schedule:** A plan to use as your weekly schedule or as a stepping stone for your own practice schedule.
- **Drills:** Each drill includes a title, category, the number of players needed and notes on how to set up the players on the court, instructions on how to run the drill, a drill diagram, and cue words that you can use during the drill to better help your players grow.
- **REC+ Factor:** Drills with the REC+ Factor have variations designed to challenge players or teams that are at a more advanced level.
- **Worksheets:** Scan and print copies of these pages for each of your players to track their own progress on. The worksheets, found at the back of the book, are integrated into the weekly practice schedules as a way to challenge your players and track their progress during practice or on their own at home.
- **Quick Lessons:** Quick descriptions of how to teach skills needed for practice.
- **Quick Drills:** Simple drills that don't need diagrams or long explanations; these are integrated into practice schedules for easy transitions between other lessons and drills.
- **Volleyball Glossary:** Helpful cue words and phrases used throughout the curriculum with a deeper explanation of the term or how it works.
- **Troubleshooting Manual:** A simple way to figure out what may be going wrong when a player is experiencing an issue. It offers answers as to what could be causing the error and ideas on how to correct it.
- **Fundamental Skill Progressions:** If you are ever wondering if a skill is too advanced for the level of players you are working with, you can refer to the Fundamental Skill Progressions. If the skill has an X in that level's column, it is an appropriate skill to teach to that age. If not, the skill may be too advanced for that level and there could be a better way to spend time in practice.
- **Drill Index:** A list of all drills in the Youth Volleyball Curriculum, organized by type. A helpful reference guide if you are looking for a specific type of drill for practice.

Drill Key

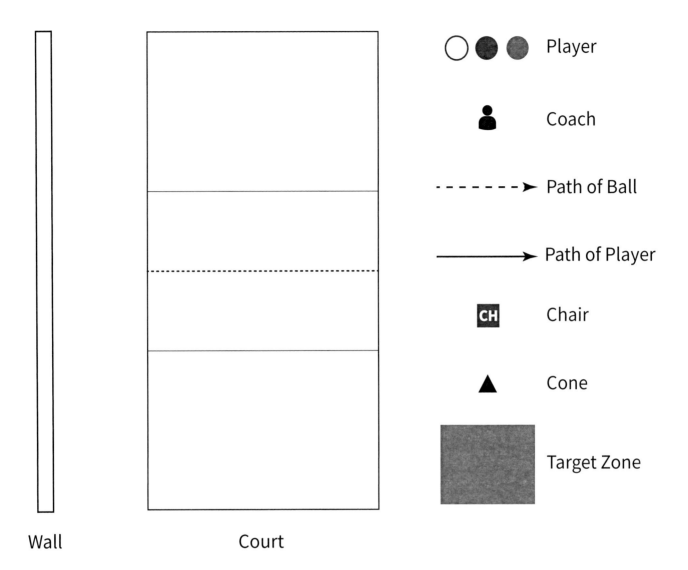

Wall   Court

○ ● ●   Player

👤   Coach

– – – – – ►   Path of Ball

——————►   Path of Player

CH   Chair

▲   Cone

Target Zone

Year One

Year One is about playing with the volleyball and having fun while learning about movements found throughout the game. Teaching stopping on a hop, running to a stop, and changing from overhead striking to a wide base are examples of these age-appropriate movements.

Practice Schedule
Year One

	Page	Drill
Week 5	9	Early Bird Special
	19	Hips to the Ball
	15	Patterns
	250	Ball Slaps
	20	Volleyball Tennis
	18	Red, White, and Blue Hitting
	21	Chair Passing
	22	Team Popcorn
Week 6	239	Sticker Chart
	240	Personal Best Score Card (Year 1-3)
	23	Serves to Wall
Week 7		**Game Week**
	9	Early Bird Special
	251	Tennis Ball Wall Throws
	24	Queens of the Court
	25	Jail Break
	26	Touchdown Serves
Week 8	9	Early Bird Special
	27	Volleyball Jog
	19	Hips to the Ball
	18	Red, White, and Blue Hitting
	16	Mock Serving
	240	Personal Best Score Card (Year 1-3)
	25	Jail Break
Week 9	9	Early Bird Special
	27	Volleyball Jog
	28	Wall Work Series
	240	Personal Best Score Card (Year 1-3)

Year 1

Spot Tossing and Thumbs Up Catching
Passing Drill

Number of Players: Partners

Player Positions: Net to Baseline

Instructions

One partner stands on the baseline of the court ("the passer") and the other partner has their back on the net ("the tosser") on the same side of the court. The tosser gives "rainbows" to the passer. The passer's goal is to move their feet to the ball and catch the ball in their mid-line (the middle of their body). The passer identifies the ball by "claiming it" and calling "My ball!" The passer should try to catch the ball with their platform extended out in front, with a hand on each side of the ball and their thumbs pointing up. Let's call that platform "long and strong."

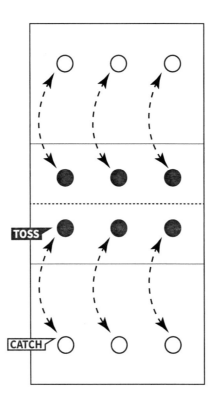

Cues

- Rainbow tosses
- Passer in ready stance
- Feet, feet, freeze
- "Claim" the ball
- Tosses short of the passer

Number of Players: All

Player Positions: Scattered

Instructions

The Early Bird Special (EBS) is all about hitting the ground running. Players get a ball immediately upon entering the gym and begin their EBS routine or the warm-up. Players stay engaged and repeat until the coach brings the full group together. The EBS should end the question, "What do we do?" as players arrive.

Year 1

Example 1

1. Jog two laps
2. 20 floor down balls
3. 20 wall sets
4. 20 self-bumps
5. 10 wall serves

Example 2

1. 25 jumping Jills
2. 5 push ups
3. 20 wall serves
4. Pepper with a pal

Example 3

1. 50 popcorns
2. 50 self-sets
3. 50 down balls

Example 4

1. 20 net jumps
2. 30 partner passes and sets
3. 40 line runs

Cues

– Same or different challenges
– Serves as you warm-up
– Reviews and reinforces skills
– Immediate touches

Team Circle Passing
Passing Drill

Number of Players: Groups of Five or Six   **Player Positions:** Groups in Circles

Instructions

From a circle formation, players start with a toss and begin passing, setting, or a combination of both to other members of the circle while counting the number of consecutive bumps or sets. Once the ball falls to the floor, the circle starts over. The circle may compete with another for a certain amount of time. This is a great drill for players after returning to the floor after a drink.

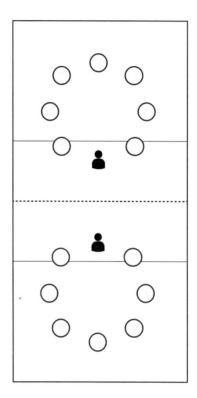

Cues

- Toss comes from coach to ensure equal opportunities
- Pass or set for personal best
- A dropped attempt ends the rally
- Circles can compete in a timed round
- Communicate using names
- All stay low, low, low
- High passes and sets buy time
- "It's up!"

Toss, Claim, Catch
Passing Drill

Number of Players: Partners

Player Positions: Partners Across Net

Instructions

Players have a partner across the net. With a slap the tosser says, "It's up!" and tosses the ball over the net. The receiver shuffles to get their hips to the ball and catches with a long and strong platform. The ultimate goal is claiming the ball by calling "My ball, my ball!" before the ball gets over the net. Young players very new to the game believe you call the ball as it contacts the platform, so calling the ball before is usually a new challenge.

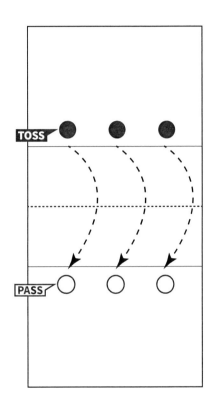

Cues

– Passers in ready stance
– Claim, "My Ball," before toss crosses the plane of the net
– Claim, don't blame!
– Catch the ball before it hits the ground
– Feet-feet freeze
– Hips to the ball
– **Goal:** early claim

Inked Up
Passing Lesson

Number of Players: All　　　　　　　　**Player Positions:** Circled Around Coach

Instructions

Asking permission to Ink Up will leave players with a thumbs together platform and long and strong arms. When the players thumbs are together the coach will draw a complete "smile" across both thumbs using a washable marker. One dot on each thumb makes the two eye dots. Two eyes makes the smile happy! Two long lines are put on the passer's platform to create a "pink zone" to later be checked, this zone is the ideal ball contact area.

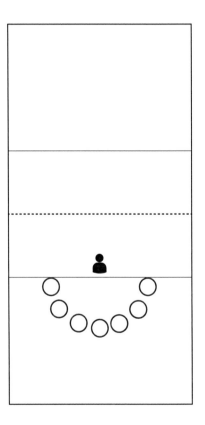

Cues

- Happy smile keeps that platform "happy"
- Long and strong
- Thumbs to the floor
- Bat thumbs: back of the thumbs together

Number of Players: All

Player Positions: Circles

Instructions

Players learn to individually control the ball by "popping," passing to themselves. The quick punch or pop right before contact is the goal. Players have fun alternating their popcorn or by seeing how many consecutive popcorn contacts they can complete. Coaches can add to the challenge by adding the one-two-cross, meaning two contacts on one arm and pop it over to two contacts on the other. Remind players to have their hips behind their heels in an active, athletic stance. Also, do not reach for the ball but shuffle over with active feet.

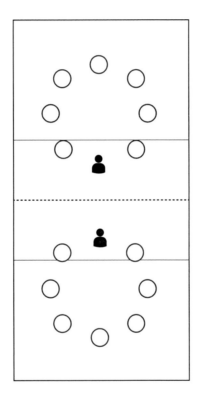

Cues

– Active feet
– Athletic stance
– Be vocal, count out loud

Air Popcorn Machine
Ball Control Drill

Number of Players: All   **Player Positions:** One Large Circle

Instructions

Players circle up and each start to popcorn individually. Once a ball hits the floor it's out but the player stays in. Coach can help control the drill by adding volleyballs back into the drill from a toss, so the Air Popcorn Machine is always working! There really is no winning or losing with this drill, the goal is to simply keeping the popcorn up and the machine running.

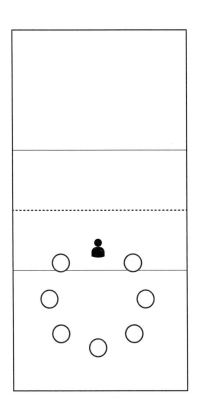

Cues

– All have a ball
– Be active
– Feet, feet, freeze
– **Communicate:** "Go, Go, Go!," "My Ball"
– **Goal:** keep the popcorn popping
– **Challenge:** add more volleyballs

Number of Players: All

Player Positions: Scattered

Instructions

Coach yells out, "Popcorn, popcorn," "Self-set, self-set," etc and players all attempt that challenge of patterns. A pattern might be, "down ball, popcorn, self-set" or perhaps, "self-set, popcorn." Players can partner up and give one another a pattern and the coach has to guess your creative ball handling pattern.

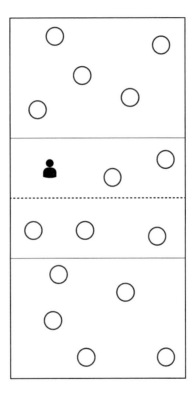

Year 1

Commands

– Floor down balls
– Popcorn
– Self-sets
– Call out "The Pattern!"

Mock Serving
Serving Drill

Number of Players: Partners   **Player Positions:** Partners Across Net

Instructions

Partners are across the net from one another starting at the 10' line. The receiving partner is a big target with hands up, ready to catch. Serving partner is focused on the details of serving as coach places emphasis and reminders on the toss, the ball alignment, the punch, etc. Players are asked to take one step back after a few minutes of serving.

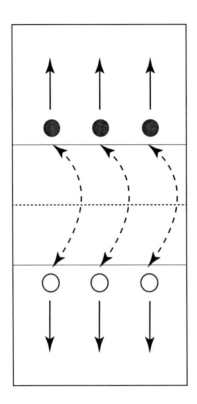

Cues

Overhand:
- Toss, step, punch
- Elbow by the eye
- Finish firm

Underhand:
- Ball on shoulder
- Drip of sweat
- 1, 2, punch

Number of Players: All　　　　　　**Player Positions:** Three Lines on Baseline

Instructions

With three lines on the baseline (3LoBL), this coach-toss drill is fast moving! Coach slaps every ball, yelling, "It's up!" as players shuffle hips to the ball and pass to the setter's zone. After passing, the passer runs up to the setter's zone to catch or put the ball in the cart. Players return to their lines after passing, setting or catching, and shagging a ball. If the pass is not catchable the setter still goes and gets it so the drill can be fluid.

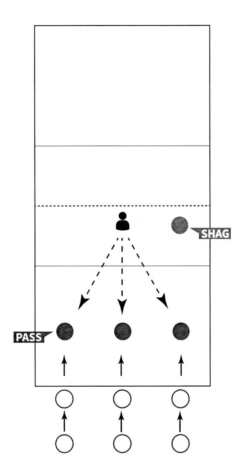

Cues

– Feet, feet, freeze
– Hips to the ball
– "Shovel" the pass
– Communicate

Red, White, and Blue Hitting
Hitting Drill

Number of Players: All   **Player Positions:** Three Lines on Baseline

Instructions

This basic striking drill is about ball alignment on the hitting shoulder and learning to hit with an open hand. Players must ask for the ball by yelling, "Red, red, red!," "White, white, white!" or "Blue, blue, blue!" Once the coach hears them calling for the ball, the coach tosses a high toss. Players shuffle to get their shoulder lined up with the ball, point with their off-hand to the ball (track), and get into the trophy top pose. Stepping with the opposite foot and smacking the ball should be complete with a "firm finish," the statue pose at the end where the player is not falling off balance after contact.

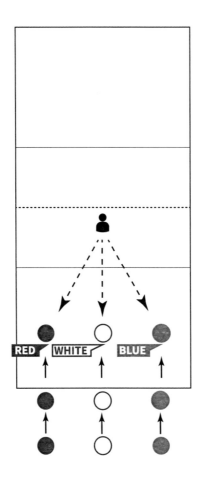

Cues

– Shoulder on ball
– High elbow
– Reach
– Trophy top
– Track and smack
– Finish firm

Number of Players: Groups of Three

Player Positions: Lines of Three

Instructions

As the tossers roll the ball back and forth, the passer shuffles using one or two shuffles or a shuffle-hop to get frozen prior to the ball reaching their stance. The ball travels through the passers feet and after a few minutes, the coach has players rotate by asking for a new player in the middle. The goal is to maintain a wide, athletic stance.

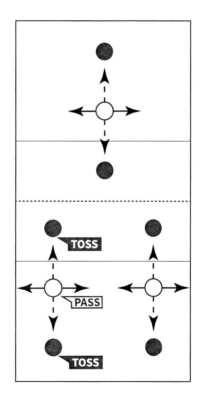

Cues

– Shuffles to alignment
– Ball travels through player's stance
– Feet, feet, freeze
– Hips to ball

Volleyball Tennis
Passing Drill

Number of Players: Partners   **Player Positions:** Net to Baseline

Instructions

Spacial awareness to the ball is our goal. Players learn to position their hips to the ball while distancing themselves from the volleyball. An open-close-open platform teaches players to move with their hands apart and place them together before contacting the ball. One partner, with their back on the net - a step or two in is fine, and the other partner a step or so in from the baseline allows partners to toss back and forth. The one bounce can get a little tougher as the drill moves along.

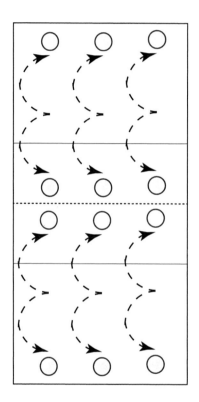

Cues

- Starts with a toss
- One bounce
- Distance from the ball
- Feet, feet, freeze
- Open-close-open platform

Number of Players: Groups of Three

Player Positions: Lines of Three

Instructions

This is a three player drill. Players are positioned with the tosser in the middle, facing the passer, and the setter or target with their back on the net. From coach's whistle, the ball is slapped and after the passer calls "It's up," the tosser tosses to the passer. The passer then bumps the ball all the way up to the setter or target. The setter simply catches the ball on their forehead in the setter's window and gently tosses it back to the tosser. On the coaches call the players will rotate in the pattern or flight the ball traveled, ie: Tosser goes to Passer, Passer goes to Setter, Setter rotates to Tosser.

Year 1

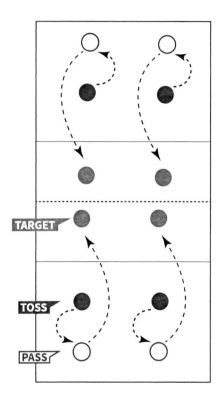

Cues

– Passers "shovel" or "shrug" to target, no swing
– Shoulders to ears
– Alligator finish

Team Popcorn
Passing Drill

Number of Players: All   **Player Positions:** Scattered on One Side

Instructions

The drill is a communication drill that has all players staying disciplined to a specific area or zone on the floor. The entire team is on one side of the net. The coach is positioned across on the other side of the net. Coach quickly puts up one toss after another over the net as players communicate, identify, claim and pass the volleyball up to the setter's zone. The goal might be a number of consecutive touches or that no ball hits the floor in 30 seconds (timed).

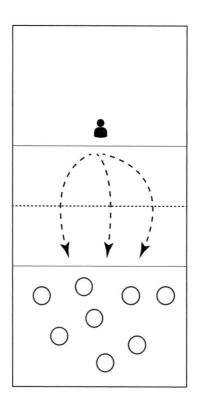

Cues

- **Coach:** rapid tossing
- **Timed:** 30 seconds
- Communicate and claim
- Stay low
- Be ready for the next ball

Number of Players: All

Player Positions: Facing Wall

Instructions

Players wall serve while being timed, as a team. Every time a serve successfully contacts the wall above the drawn on or taped line the player yells out the next count. For example, one player serves above the line and they yells, "One!" Several serves later another player serves successfully and they yells out "Two!" Players set a Team Personal Best and try to beat their own score in a second or third attempt. One minute on the clock and go!

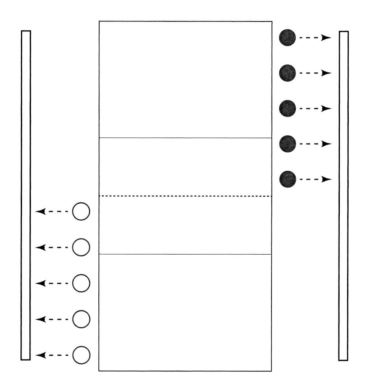

Cues

- **Timed:** One minute
- Rapid serving and counting
- Ball to shoulder
- Fast hips
- Open and close
- Elbow by the eye
- Finish firm

Queens of the Court
Team Drill

Number of Players: All   **Player Positions:** Three Lines on Baseline

Instructions

Players line up in three lines on the baseline while coach is across the net from the Queen side with a cart of volleyballs. First player in each line are the Queens (Q). As the Queens dip under the net to find the Royal Courtyard, the Princesses (P) step on to challenge them. The coach always tosses across the net to the Queen side. If either side attempts three hits by passing a controlled pass up to the setter's zone, the coach grants a life and that team gets a "do over." A life is a way to emphasize three hits volleyball. When a play ends, new Challengers (CH) come onto the floor and either the Queens remain (Queens won the point) or new Queens run under the net to take over (Princesses won the point). Whichever side lost the point always shags the volleyball and returns to their lines. For an uneven number of players encourage new partners.

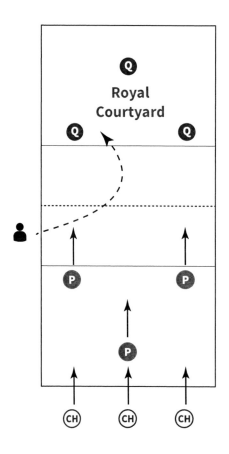

Cues

– Queens receive ball
– Call, "Free ball!" on coach's slap
– **Earn a life:** pass goes to setter zone
– **Queens win point:** Queens stay, Challengers step on
– **Princesses win point:** Queens off, Princesses move to Queen side, Challengers step on

Number of Players: All

Player Positions: Service Line

Instructions

All players serve from the Law Abiding Citizens side of the net. When a serve is missed the player who missed is "off to jail." There are two ways a player can get out of jail: coach yells "Jail break!" or a player claims a serve and catches it. If a player catches the volleyball from jail, they go back to the serving side and the player whose ball was caught goes to jail! This classic drill is always a team favorite.

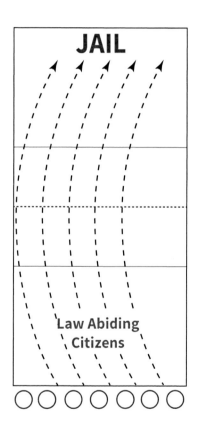

Cues

- Routine to punch
- **Good serve:** keep serving
- **Miss:** off to jail
- **Ticket out of jail:** catch a served ball
- **Serve is caught:** off to jail
- Coach may call "Jail break!" to free all

Touchdown Serves
Serving Drill

Number of Players: All   **Player Positions:** Servers on Wall

Instructions

From a complete routine, for example: two-dribbles, step back, cool spin, one-two-punch, players work hard as individuals or small teams to score a football field goal! Coach tapes large uprights, depending on age or challenge level wanted, on the wall for players to serve with accuracy. Remember coaches to get those uprights high. When a player gets a serve through the uprights, they yell, "TOUCHDOWN (and their favorite team)!"

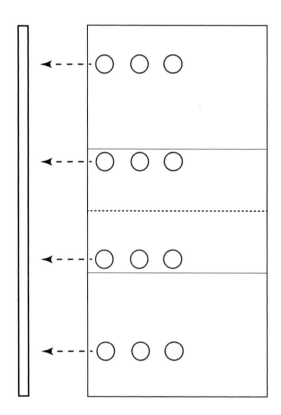

Cues

Overhand:
– Toss, step, punch
– Elbow by the eye
– Finish firm

Underhand:
– Ball on shoulder
– Drip of sweat
– 1, 2, punch

– Players yell "Touchdown!" when the ball goes through the uprights.

Number of Players: All

Player Positions: Around Court

Instructions

The players go for a light and easy jog around the floor - as a team! With a ball under their arm, players stop on coaches whistle and as they "rest" they perform a series of ball handling challenges such as popcorn, down balls, and self-sets. Once a challenge is over, players go another lap or two awaiting the whistle for their next task. This is a good ball handling activity.

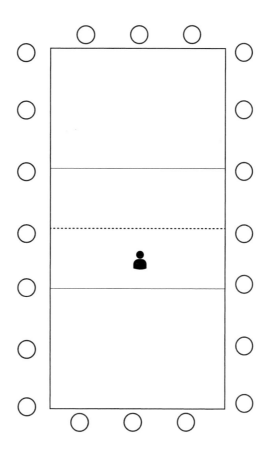

Cues

– Team jogs around the court
– Big and soft hands when setting
– Long and strong arms when passing

Coach stops team to perform challenges:

– Popcorn
– Self-sets
– Low passing catches
– Floor down balls

Wall Work Series
Ball Control Drill

Number of Players: All   **Player Positions:** On Wall

Instructions

Wall work is for individual player development. Players find an area on the wall and move through a series of skills including: wall sets, wall down balls from a knee, wall down balls from standing, serving wall pins, serving wall deliveries or steady serving tosses, wall passing, and full wall serves , stepping off the wall 15-20 feet. This series can range from 30 seconds to 2 minutes per skill set.

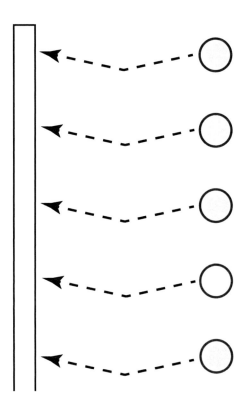

Drills

– Sets
– Down balls from knee
– Down balls standing
– Pins
– Tosses, shoulder on line
– Passes
– Serves

Year Two

Year Two graduates from balloons, nerf balls, and noodles, which are still fun, to more consistent and volleyball-like touches using a smaller beach ball and light volleyballs. Building on their striking skills is important along with learning to get their hands together in their platform before the ball falls. Reaction time to the ball and repetition with movement and striking are key for early success. Success, of course, being defined as kids having fun and loving volleyball!

Much can be taught to this age group "off the bounce" as young players learn to time the rebound bounce and their contact. Shuffling to the ball and agility challenges are helpful while building on their volleyball vocabulary, adding terms to match cue words and phrases. For example, rocking chair feet, meaning transfer of weight.

Practice Schedule
Year Two

	Page	Drill
Week 5	36	Early Bird Special
	250	Partner Tossing
	251	Wall Down balls from knees or standing
	32	Popcorn Series
	45	Jail break
	48	Spider Web
	251	Challenge: 30 Wall Bumps and Sets
Week 6	36	Early Bird Special
	251	Wall Down Balls
	250	10-5-1 Wall Challenge
	37	Juggling Patterns
	240	Personal Best Score Card (Year 1-3)
	231	10 Team Serves
	246	Lesson: Free Ball
	49	Queens of the Court
Week 7	36	Early Bird Special
	50	Patterns
	51	Volleyball Jog
	250	10-5-1 Wall Challenge
	43	Red, White, and Blue Hitting
	52	Shuffle,Shuffle,Freeze "Dance"
	53	Net Down Balls
	54	Coach's Passing
	55	Pass One, Hit One, Combo
	56	Challenge: Team Circle Passing and Setting
Week 8	36	Early Bird Special
	250	Partner Passing
	240	Personal Best Score Card (Year 1-3)
	239	Sticker Chart
	45	Jail Break
Week 9	36	Early Bird Special
	32	Popcorn Series
	37	Patterns
	57	3 LoBL Combo Touches
	49	Queens of the Court

Year 2

Popcorn Series
Ball Control Drill

Number of Players: All   **Player Positions:** Circles

Instructions

Players learn to individually control the ball by "popping," passing to themselves. The quick punch or pop right before contact is the goal. Players have fun alternating their popcorn or by seeing how many consecutive popcorn contacts they can complete. Coaches can add to the challenge by adding the one-two-cross, meaning two contacts on one arm and pop it over to two contacts on the other. Remind players to have their hips behind their heels in an active, athletic stance. Also, do not reach for the ball but shuffle over with active feet.

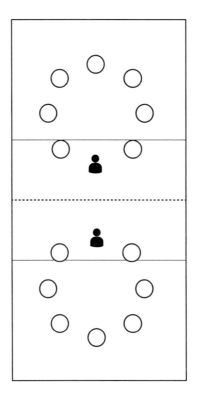

Cues

- Active feet
- Athletic stance
- Be vocal, count out loud

Number of Players: All　　　　　　**Player Positions:** Two Lines on Baseline

Instructions

The Target Spots are either large free ball areas (FB) across the net from the players or a designated setter's zone (SZ) on the same side of the net. With two lines of passers and a coach-toss formation, coach can either call out a zone or players attempt a controlled pass to zone or an aggressive free ball to the large area across the net. Note: players should have two different looks as they adjust to the ball or skill; hips to the ball, frozen passing or a free-ball stance, hips to the sideline, and shoulder closest to the net dropped for an aggressive free ball.

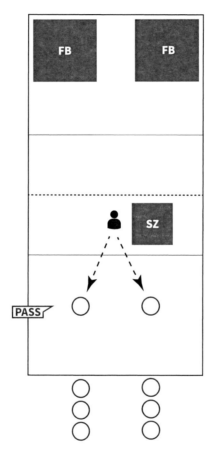

Cues

Player Strive to Get the Ball to Target:
– Pass: aiming for setter's zone (SZ)
– Free ball: aiming for free ball zones (FB)

Different Body Posture:
– Passing: hips to the ball, frozen passing
– Free balling: hips to the sideline, shoulder dropped

Spot Tossing and Thumbs Up Catching
Passing Drill

Number of Players: Partners

Player Positions: Net to Baseline

Instructions

One partner stands on the baseline of the court ("the passer") and the other partner has their back on the net ("the tosser") on the same side of the court. The tosser gives "rainbows" to the passer. The passer's goal is to move their feet to the ball and catch the ball in their mid-line (the middle of their body). The passer identifies the ball by "claiming it" and calling "My ball!" The passer should try to catch the ball with their platform extended out in front, with a hand on each side of the ball and their thumbs pointing up. Let's call that platform "long and strong."

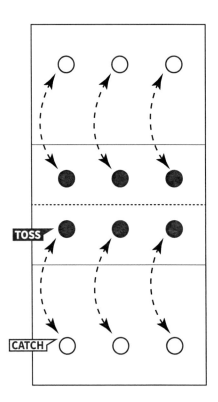

Cues

- Rainbow tosses
- Passer in ready stance
- Feet, feet, freeze
- "Claim" the ball
- Tosses short of the passer

Number of Players: All

Player Positions: Scattered

Instructions

Players individually toss very high and let the ball bounce once. Players draw their hands above their head to create a setter's window for catching with "setter's hands," or players show patience in letting the ball fall very close to the floor before catching it with "passer's feet, arms, and hands," thumbs up on sides of volleyball. Coach can call out challenge or players can alternate skills. Have players check their feet as much as their hands and platform.

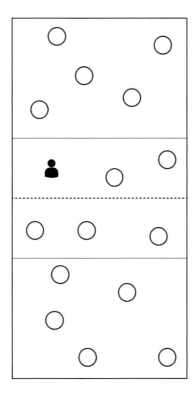

Cues

Passing: players toss high, let the ball bounce once and catch low
- Thumbs up
- Platform long and strong
- Lengthen and extend

Setting: players toss high, let the ball bounce once and catch high
- Arms up fast
- Hands above your head
- Setting window

Early Bird Special
Warm-up Drill

Number of Players: All

Player Positions: Scattered

Instructions

The Early Bird Special (EBS) is all about hitting the ground running. Players get a ball immediately upon entering the gym and begin their EBS routine or the warm-up. Players stay engaged and repeat until the coach brings the full group together. The EBS should end the question, "what do we do?" as players arrive.

Example 1

1. Jog two laps
2. 20 floor down balls
3. 20 wall sets
4. 20 self-bumps
5. 10 wall serves

Example 2

1. 25 jumping Jills
2. 5 push ups
3. 20 wall serves
4. Pepper with a pal

Example 3

1. 50 popcorns
2. 50 self-sets
3. 50 down balls

Example 4

1. 20 net jumps
2. 30 partner passes and sets
3. 40 line runs

Cues

– Same or different challenges
– Serves as you warm-up
– Reviews and reinforces skills
– Immediate touches

Number of Players: All

Player Positions: Scattered

Instructions

Coach calls out a series of ball handling challenges. Coach may request a pattern of these challenges or a series. For example, coach yells out - "20 self-sets followed by 20 self bumps." The goal is to have ball control and numerous, fast touches.

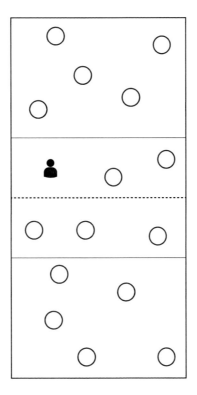

Cues

– Claim the ball
– Keep the ball in your own area

Challenges:

– Self bumps
– Self-sets
– Sand pokies
– Floor down balls

Four Muscle Memory Throws
Warm-up Drill

Number of Players: Partners

Player Positions: Net to Baseline

Instructions

There are four muscle-memory throws:

1) Two Thumbs by the Thighs - players, positioned with a partner, throw for warm-up and also for developing essential movements in overhand serving, hitting, and hip rotation. Two Thumbs by the Thighs has partners bouncing the ball hard once to the floor - playing catch - back and forth.

2) Elbow by the Eye - players pause and adjust their throwing arm to get the throwing arm elbow "by the eye." As they throw with the opposite foot forward, the coach reminds players of the **opening and closing** of their hips. Players throw from **high to low**, meaning wrist snap at the release, aiming for the receiving partners knee pads.

3) Back to Your Partner - partners face away from their partner and step forward, with either foot to switch it up, arching the back and "throwing their chest to the ceiling" and holding their arms way up high pose.

4) Two Slaps and a Down Ball - two big open hand "slappy" sounds on the ball followed by a down ball to their partner. The ball bounces once. Remind players in this "throw" to not toss the ball but hit it out of their own hand or after a very small toss.

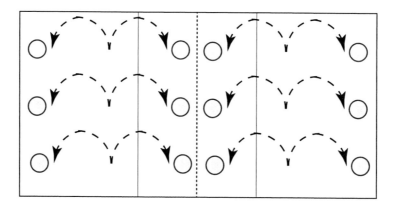

Cues

Throws:

1) Two Thumbs by the Thigh	Hard throws to the floor
2) Elbow by the Eye	Elbow starts high and leads
3) Back to Your Partner	Big and animated
4) Two Slaps and a Down Ball	Slaps with elbow lead

Number of Players: All   **Player Positions:** Lines

Instructions

The team is in lines, orderly and uniform. As the coach moves players through a series of static stretches the players stay involved and engaged by counting and holding the stretches. The coach yells out the **odd** numbers as the players count the **even** numbers. Players either clap two times or slap the floor two times after the 10 count and chant their team name!

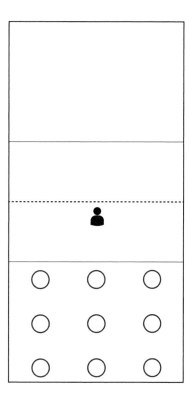

Suggested Stretches:

– RT over LT
– LT over RT
– Straddle
– Arm front and behind stretches
– Butterfly and hurdle stretch

Rainbow Tosses
Passing Drill

Number of Players: Partners

Player Positions: Partners Across Net

Instructions

Players are positioned across the net from one another. Learning to control a two-hand toss from a wide base, thumbs up with a high delivery will be complete when players toss **short** of their receiver. Use tape, dots, hula hoops, or a cone to identify the ideal area for the ball to drop in. Passers or receivers should be down in the ready position, practicing claiming the ball, and catching the ball with long and strong arms.

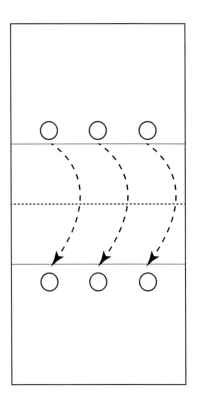

Cues

– Feet, feet, freeze
– Long and strong
– Distance from the ball
– Claim the ball

Number of Players: Groups of Three

Player Positions: Lines of Three

Instructions

As the tossers roll the ball back and forth, the passer shuffles using one or two shuffles or a shuffle-hop to get frozen prior to the ball reaching their stance. The ball travels through the passers feet and after a few minutes, the coach has players rotate by asking for a new player in the middle. The goal is to be frozen before the ball travels through the players stance and maintain a wide, athletic stance.

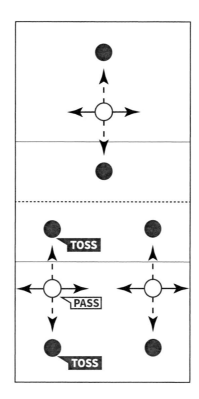

Cues

– Shuffles to alignment
– Ball travels through player's stance
– Feet, feet, freeze
– Hips to ball

Team Popcorn
Passing Drill

Number of Players: All   **Player Positions:** Scattered on One Side

Instructions

The drill is a communication drill that has all players staying disciplined to a specific area or zone on the floor. The entire team is on one side of the net. The coach is positioned across on the other side of the net. Coach quickly puts up one toss after another over the net as players communicate, identify, claim and pass the volleyball up to the setter's zone. The goal might be a number of consecutive touches or that no ball hits the floor in 30 seconds (timed).

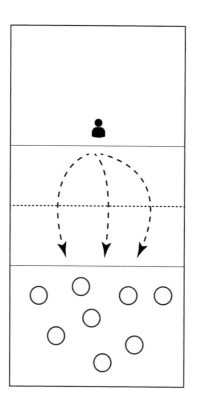

Cues

– **Coach:** rapid tossing
– **Timed:** 30 seconds
– Communicate and claim
– Stay low
– Be ready for the next ball

Red, White, and Blue Hitting
Hitting Drill

Number of Players: All

Player Positions: Three Lines on Baseline

Instructions

This basic striking drill is about ball alignment on the hitting shoulder and learning to hit with an open hand. Players must ask for the ball by yelling, "Red, red, red!," "White, white, white!" or "Blue, blue, blue!" Once the coach hears them calling for the ball, the coach tosses a high toss. Players shuffle to get their shoulder lined up with the ball, point with their off-hand to the ball (track), and get into the trophy top pose. Stepping with the opposite foot and smacking the ball should be complete with a "firm finish," the statue pose at the end where the player is not falling off balance after contact.

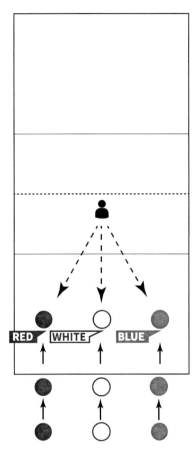

Year 2

Cues

– Shoulder on ball
– High elbow
– Reach
– Trophy top
– Track and smack
– Finish firm

Mock Serving
Serving Drill

Number of Players: Partners   **Player Positions:** Partners Across Net

Instructions

Partners are across the net from one another starting at the 10' line. The receiving partner is a big target with hands up, ready to catch. Serving partner is focused on the details of serving as coach places emphasis and reminders on the toss, the ball alignment, the punch, etc. Players are asked to take one step back after a few minutes of serving.

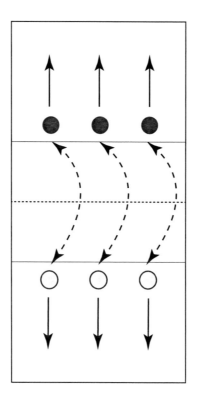

Cues

Overhand:
– Toss, step, punch
– Elbow by the eye
– Finish firm

Underhand:
– Ball on shoulder
– Drip of sweat
– 1, 2, punch

Number of Players: All

Player Positions: Service Line

Instructions

All players serve from the Law Abiding Citizens side of the net. When a serve is missed the player who missed is "off to jail." There are two ways a player can get out of jail: coach yells "Jail break!" or a player claims a serve and catches it. If a player catches the volleyball from jail, they go back to the serving side and the player whose ball was caught goes to jail! This classic drill is always a team favorite.

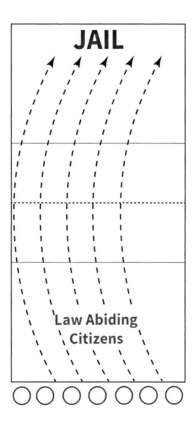

Cues

- Routine to punch
- **Good serve:** keep serving
- **Miss:** off to jail
- **Ticket out of jail:** catch a served ball
- **Serve is caught:** off to jail
- Coach may call "Jail break!" to free all

Dynamic Warm-up
Warm-up Drill

Number of Players: All   **Player Positions:** Three Lines on Baseline

Instructions

Dynamic warm-up includes a series of stretches from high knees to bottom kicks. Players line up in three lines on the baseline and on the coach's whistle are brought out from their lines. Players can do the warm-up exercise to the net and back, with lots of high-fives and enthusiasm as they return to the line. Coach can emphasize players being **attentive** and **invested** in the details and remind the players to "lift toes," "drive the knee," "keep shoulders parallel with the wall," etc.

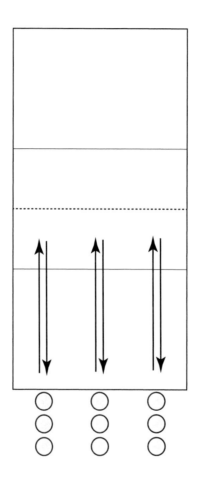

Suggested Exercises:

– High knee with a skip
– Bounds with a skip
– Butt kickers
– Grapevine
– Frankensteins
– Jogging, forwards and backwards

Number of Players: Partners

Player Positions: Passer on Wall

Instructions

The passing partner starts a few feet from the wall while the tossing partner is about 12-20 feet from the wall. The passer's challenge is to drop step and open their hips to shuffle back to the wall, touch it, and return to the passing ready position. The passer then control passes back to the tosser. The tosser must wait for the passer to touch the wall before they slap the ball with an "It's up!" call. The coach rotates players every 45 seconds to a minute. Challenge the Passer to **not stand** between passing but stay low the entire time.

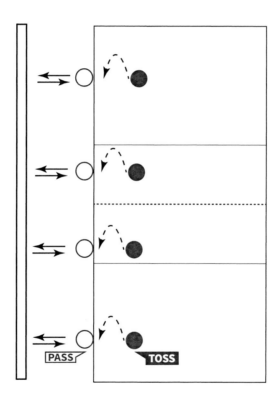

Cues

– **Passer:** "Freezes and sits" and "drops hips"
– **Tosser:** distributes short toss to approaching passer

Spiderweb
Serving Drill

Number of Players: All   **Player Positions:** Scattered on Half the Floor

Instructions

All volleyball players report to the spiderweb! The web is on one side of the floor anywhere inbounds but behind the 10' line. Coach picks a couple of "serving spiders" to begin serving the spider eggs (volleyballs) over the net into the web full of spiders. When a serving spider hits a spider directly, that spider becomes a serving spider. Make sure players are facing the serving spiders and they cover their heads if a spider egg looks like it's going to hit them above the shoulders. When all spiders are serving and the game is down to the last two or three spiders, the non-serving spiders become the new serving spiders, starting a new game. Spiders cannot move unless the coach yells out "Spider shuffle!" then the spiders all jump up, dance the spider dance, and return to the web after the serving spiders go shag all the volleyballs - of course, we mean spider eggs!

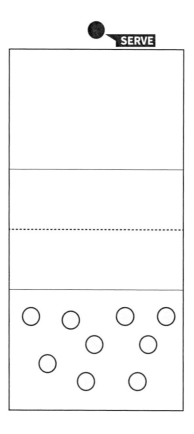

Cues

- **Goal:** have all spiders serving to get that last spider
- A direct hit "frees" the hit spider to serve
- Do not allow the spiders to be in front of the 10 ft line

Number of Players: All

Player Positions: Three Lines on Baseline

Instructions

Players line up in three lines on the baseline while coach is across the net from the Queen side with a cart of volleyballs. First player in each line are the Queens (Q). As the Queens dip under the net to find the Royal Courtyard, the Princesses (P) step on to challenge them. The coach always tosses across the net to the Queen side. If either side attempts three hits by passing a controlled pass up to the setter's zone, the coach grants a life and that team gets a "do over." A life is a way to emphasize three hits volleyball. When a play ends, new Challengers (CH) come onto the floor and either the Queens remain (Queens won the point) or new Queens run under the net to take over (Princesses won the point). Whichever side lost the point always shags the volleyball and returns to their lines. For an uneven number of players encourage new partners.

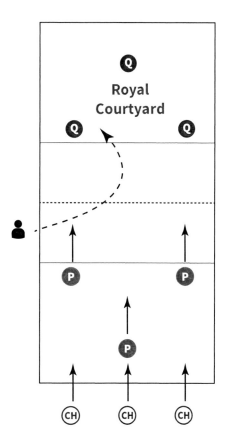

Cues

– Queens receive ball
– Call, "Free ball!" on coach's slap
– **Earn a life:** pass goes to setter zone
– **Queens win point:** Queens stay, Challengers step on
– **Princesses win point:** Queens off, Princesses move to Queen side, Challengers step on

Patterns
Ball Control Drill

Number of Players: All

Instructions

Coach yells out, "popcorn, popcorn, self-set, self-set" and players all attempt that challenge of patterns. A pattern might be, "down ball, popcorn, self-set" or perhaps, "self-set, popcorn." Players can partner up and give one another a pattern and the coach has to guess your creative ball handling pattern.

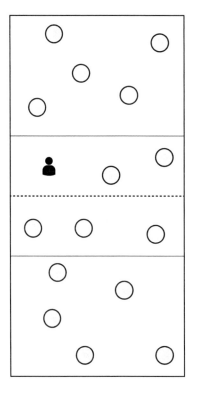

Commands

– Floor down balls
– Popcorn
– Self-sets
– Call out "The Pattern!"

Number of Players: All

Player Positions: Around Court

Instructions

The players go for a light and easy jog around the floor - as a team! With a ball under their arm, players stop on coaches whistle and as they "rest" they perform a series of ball handling challenges such as popcorn, down balls, and self-sets. Once a challenge is over, players go another lap or two awaiting the whistle for their next task. This is a good ball handling activity.

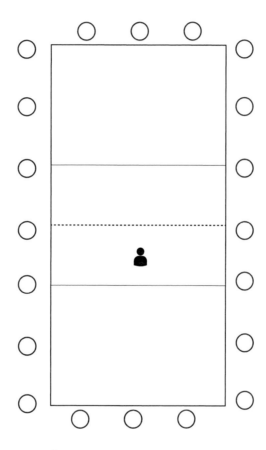

Cues

– Team jogs around the court
– Big and soft hands when setting
– Long and strong arms when passing

Coach stops team to perform challenges:

– Popcorn
– Self-sets
– Low passing catches
– Floor down balls

Shuffle, Shuffle, Freeze "Dance"
Passing Drill

Number of Players: All   **Player Positions:** Evenly Spaced

Instructions

Players are positioned in a group formation in lines, with plenty of room. Like a team dance, players follow the coaches lead and call out the footwork. Players move together in a rhythm going six to eight different directions. The coach can define the directions prior to beginning. Players must stay low and get through the six to eight spots and recover back to the middle each time. Remember coaches to face the net or have your back to the players so they can truly mirror your moves.

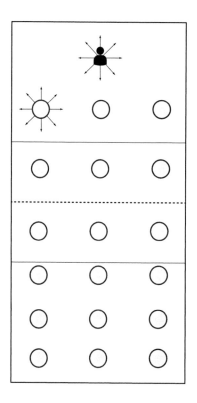

Cues

- "Dance" starts in ready stance on whistle
- Coach points the pattern and leads players in saying, "Feet, feet, freeze!" or "1, 2, freeze!"

REC+ Factor: Add a simulated movement of passing or setting at the completion of each footwork pattern.

Number of Players: Partners

Player Positions: Partners Across Net

Instructions

Partners face one another from 10' line to 10' line. Start a full step in toward the net and begin hitting down ball so that the ball bounces once **under** the net to the other partner. Players back up on cue from the coach. Players are learning where and how to strike the ball to adjust its rebound. More advanced players can attempt to put top-spin on the hits.

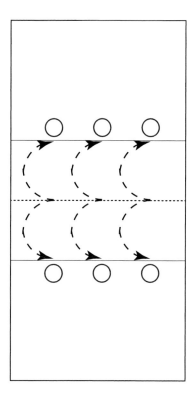

Cues

- Players down ball **under** the net back and forth
- Controlled swing, trying to hit the top of the ball
- Wrist snap
- Contact on "top third" of the ball

Coach's Passing
Passing Drill

Number of Players: All   **Player Positions:** Three Lines on Baseline

Instructions

With 3 Lines on the Baseline (3LoBL), this coach-toss drill is fast moving! Coach slaps every ball, yelling, "It's up!" as players shuffle hips to the ball and pass to the setter's zone. After passing, the passer runs up to the setter's zone to catch or put the ball in the cart. Players return to their lines after passing, setting or catching, and shagging a ball. If the pass is not catchable the setter still goes and gets it so the drill can be fluid.

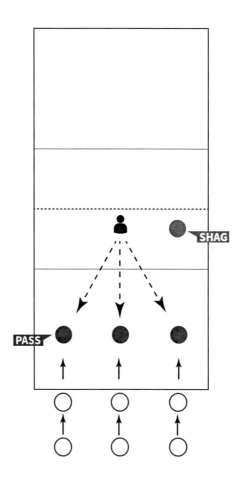

Cues

– Feet, feet, freeze
– Hips to the ball
– "Shovel" the pass
– Communicate

er Positions: Three Lines on Baseline

back. The first toss is a pass. Then, the player
own ball. The player shags two volleyballs to
eat deal of emphasis on this combination of
and efficient change with footwork, posture,

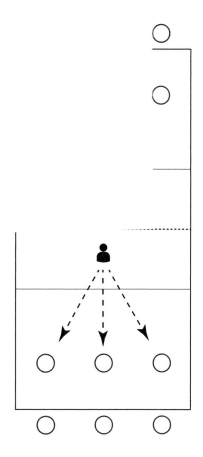

Cues

- First contact is a controlled pass
- Second is a strong hit
- Coach can reverse the order, hit then pass
- Player claims the ball when passing, "My ball, my ball!," and when hitting, "Red, red, red!"
- Players need to have a mindset that can switch from controlled to aggressive

Team Circle Passing
Passing Drill

Number of Players: Groups of Five or Six

Player Positions: Groups in Circles

Instructions

From a circle formation, players start with a toss and begin passing, setting, or a combination of both to other members of the circle while counting the number of consecutive bumps or sets. Once the ball falls to the floor, the circle starts over. The circle may compete with another for a certain amount of time. This is a great drill for players after returning to the floor after a drink.

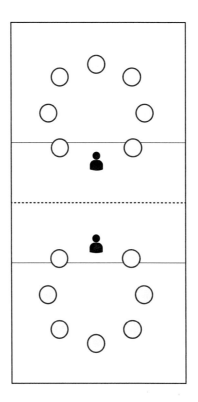

Cues

– Toss comes from coach to ensure equal opportunities
– Pass or set for personal best
– A dropped attempt ends the rally
– Circles can compete in a timed round
– Communicate using names
– All stay low, low, low
– High passes and sets buy time
– "It's up!"

Number of Players: All

Player Positions: Three Lines on Baseline

Instructions

3LoBL formation will have the first three athletes stepping into the floor. The coach communicates a series of touches or skill sets desired, for example: free ball, dig, track and smack. Players then, as a team demonstrate those skill sets in the order the coach called out. A combination of skills will determine how the coach will toss. Players are expected to call out the skill to communicate back to the coach the skill set they should be doing. Coach can emphasize some general cues throughout the drill like, frozen-feet, snap to draw setter's hands, shoulder to the ball when hitting.

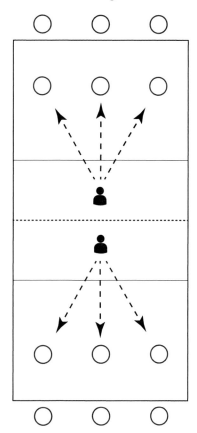

Cues

– Hip to the ball
– Fast toss
– Player call out their skill
– "Frozen feet" always priority

Coaches Commands:

– Pass
– Set
– Free ball
– Track and Smack

Year Three

Year Three players are ready to engage in tossing and simple partner challenges. Small group work and team challenges will also make their volleyball time enjoyable. Adding the "free ball" from a coach's toss over the net will enhance hand-eye coordination and teach young ones to slide over to the volleyball vs. reaching for it.

Knowing how to rotate positions and the names of each position will begin the development of the complete, academic volleyball player! Players at this age love counting! 10 self-sets, 20 jumping jacks, followed by two serves are examples of individual and large group counting and participation. This also introduces the importance of being vocal.

Year 3

Practice Schedule
Year Three

	Page	Drill
Week 6	67	Early Bird Special
	74	Baseline Throws
	240	Personal Best Score Card (Year 1-3)
	251	Wall Down Balls
	78	Queen of the Throne
	79	Volleyball Tennis
Week 7	67	Early Bird Special
	250	Partner Passing and Setting
	80	Volleyball Jog
	63	Team Stretch
	64	Four Muscle Memory Throws
	81	Shuffle, Shuffle, Freeze "Dance"
	251	Serving Wall Targets
Week 8	67	Early Bird Special
	250	Free Net Time
	63	Team Stretch
	64	Four Muscle Memory Throws
	250	Serving for Correction
	65	Popcorn Series
	68	3 Lines On Baseline Combo Touches
	251	Challenge: 20 Team Serves
Week 9	67	Early Bird Special
	251	Wall Serving and Wall Pins
	82	Three Hits Goal
	240	Personal Best Score Card (Year 1-3)
	72	Queens of the Court

Dynamic Warm-up
Warm-up Drill

Number of Players: All   **Player Positions:** Three Lines on Baseline

Instructions

Dynamic warm-up includes a series of stretches from high knees to bottom kicks. Players line up in three lines on the baseline and on the coach's whistle are brought out from their lines. Players can do the warm-up exercise to the net and back, with lots of high-fives and enthusiasm as they return to the line. Coach can emphasize players being **attentive** and **invested** in the details and remind the players to "lift toes," "drive the knee," "keep shoulders parallel with the wall," etc.

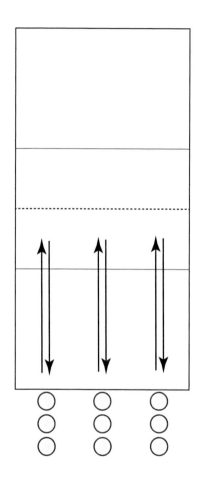

Suggested Exercises:

– High knee with a skip
– Bounds with a skip
– Butt kickers
– Grapevine
– Frankensteins
– Jogging, forwards and backwards

Number of Players: All

Player Positions: Lines

Instructions

The team is in lines, orderly and uniform. As the coach moves players through a series of static stretches the players stay involved and engaged by counting and holding the stretches. The coach yells out the **odd** numbers as the players count the **even** numbers. Players either clap two times or slap the floor two times after the 10 count and chant their team name!

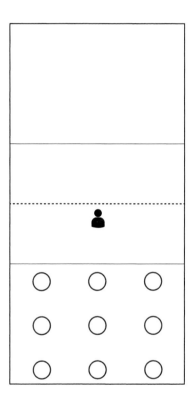

Suggested Stretches:

– RT over LT
– LT over RT
– Straddle
– Arm front and behind stretches
– Butterfly and hurdle stretch

Four Muscle Memory Throws
Warm-up Drill

Number of Players: Partners

Player Positions: Net to Baseline

Instructions

There are four muscle-memory throws:

1) Two Thumbs by the Thighs - players, positioned with a partner, throw for warm-up and also for developing essential movements in overhand serving, hitting, and hip rotation. Two Thumbs by the Thighs has partners bouncing the ball hard once to the floor - playing catch - back and forth.

2) Elbow by the Eye - players pause and adjust their throwing arm to get the throwing arm elbow "by the eye." As they throw with the opposite foot forward, the coach reminds players of the opening and closing of their hips. Players throw from high to low, meaning wrist snap at the release, aiming for the receiving partners knee pads.

3) Back to Your Partner - partners face away from their partner and step forward, with either foot to switch it up, arching the back and "throwing their chest to the ceiling" and holding their arms way up high pose.

4) Two Slaps and a Down Ball - two big open hand "slappy" sounds on the ball followed by a down ball to their partner. The ball bounces once. Remind players in this "throw" to not toss the ball but hit it out of their own hand or after a very small toss.

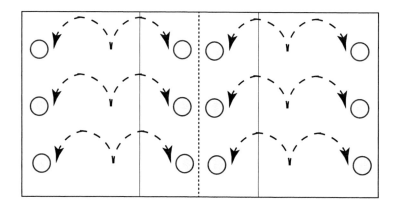

Cues

Throws:

1) Two Thumbs by the Thigh	Hard throws to the floor
2) Elbow by the Eye	Elbow starts high and leads
3) Back to Your Partner	Big and animated
4) Two Slaps and a Down Ball	Slaps with elbow lead

Number of Players: All   **Player Positions:** Circles

Instructions

Players learn to individually control the ball by "popping," passing to themselves. The quick punch or pop right before contact is the goal. Players have fun alternating their popcorn or by seeing how many consecutive popcorn contacts they can complete. Coaches can add to the challenge by adding the one-two-cross, meaning two contacts on one arm and pop it over to two contacts on the other. Remind players to have their hips behind their heels in an active, athletic stance. Also, do not reach for the ball but shuffle over with active feet.

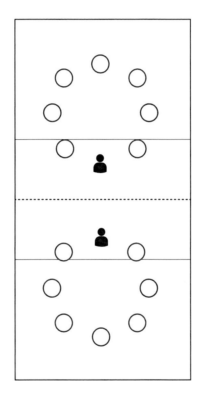

Cues

– Active feet
– Athletic stance
– Be vocal, count out loud

Team Circle Passing
Passing Drill

Number of Players: Groups of Five or Six

Player Positions: Groups in Circles

Instructions

From a circle formation, players start with a toss and begin passing, setting, or a combination of both to other members of the circle while counting the number of consecutive bumps or sets. Once the ball falls to the floor, the circle starts over. The circle may compete with another for a certain amount of time. This is a great drill for players after returning to the floor after a drink.

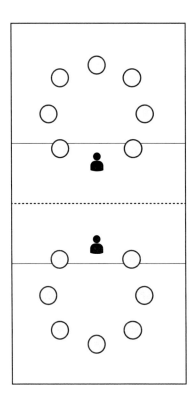

Cues

- Toss comes from coach to ensure equal opportunities
- Pass or set for personal best
- A dropped attempt ends the rally
- Circles can compete in a timed round
- Communicate using names
- All stay low, low, low
- **Reminder:** high passes and sets buy time
- "It's up!"

Early Bird Special
Warm-up Drill

Number of Players: All

Player Positions: Scattered

Instructions

The Early Bird Special (EBS) is all about hitting the ground running. Players get a ball immediately upon entering the gym and begin their EBS routine or the warm-up. Players stay engaged and repeat until the coach brings the full group together. The EBS should end the question, "what do we do?" as players arrive.

Example 1

1. Jog two laps

2. 20 floor down balls

3. 20 wall sets

4. 20 self-bumps

5. 10 wall serves

Example 2

1. 25 jumping Jills

2. 5 push ups

3. 20 wall serves

4. Pepper with a pal

Example 3

1. 50 popcorns

2. 50 self-sets

3. 50 down balls

Example 4

1. 20 net jumps

2. 30 partner passes and sets

3. 40 line runs

Year 3

Cues

– Same or different challenges
– Serves as you warm-up
– Reviews and reinforces skills
– Immediate touches

3 LoBL Combo Touches
Ball Control Drill

Number of Players: All

Player Positions: Three Lines on Baseline

Instructions

3LoBL formation will have the first three athletes stepping into the floor. The coach communicates a series of touches or skill sets desired, for example: free ball, dig, track and smack. Players then, as a team demonstrate those skill sets in the order the coach called out. A combination of skills will determine how the coach will toss. Players are expected to call out the skill to communicate back to the coach the skill set they should be doing. Coach can emphasize some general cues throughout the drill like, frozen-feet, snap to draw setter's hands, shoulder to the ball when hitting.

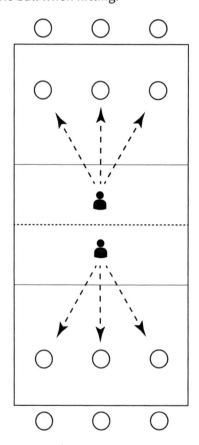

Cues

– Hip to the ball
– Fast toss
– Player call out their skill
– "Frozen feet" always priority

Coaches Commands:

– Pass
– Set
– Free ball
– Track and Smack

Pass and Set Pepper
Passing, Setting Drill

Number of Players: Partners

Player Positions: Net to Baseline

Instructions

With a partner, players are positioned one partner with their back on the net and the other on the baseline. Players will begin with a toss to their partner. From the toss the two players are challenged to keep the drill alive by "peppering," any combination of passing and setting, back and forth. Players should communicate and recover back to starting position with each contact.

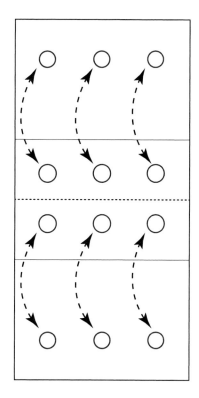

Cues

– Feet first
– Draw fast, platform last
– "1 Mississippi" hold on the follow through
–

REC+ Factor: Add a clock and personal best challenge.

Jail Break
Serving Drill

Number of Players: All

Player Positions: Service Line

Instructions

All players serve from the Law Abiding Citizens side of the net. When a serve is missed the player who missed is "off to jail." There are two ways a player can get out of jail: coach yells "Jail break!" or a player claims a serve and catches it. If a player catches the volleyball from jail, they go back to the serving side and the player whose ball was caught goes to jail! This classic drill is always a team favorite.

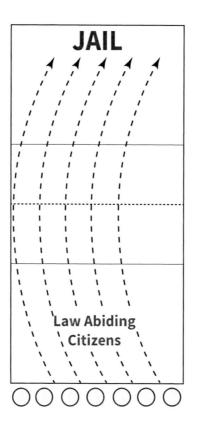

Cues

– Routine to punch
– **Good serve:** keep serving
– **Miss:** off to jail
– **Ticket out of jail:** catch a served ball
– **Serve is caught:** off to jail
– Coach may call "Jail break!" to free all

Number of Players: Partners   **Player Positions:** Partners Across Net

Instructions

Partners are across the net from one another starting at the 10' line. The receiving partner is a big target with hands up, ready to catch. Serving partner is focused on the details of serving as coach places emphasis and reminders on the toss, the ball alignment, the punch, etc. Players are asked to take one step back after a few minutes of serving.

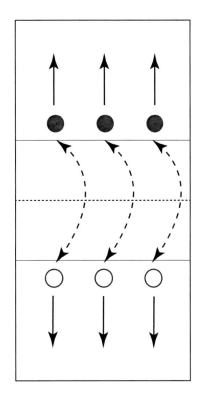

Cues

Overhand:
– Toss, step, punch
– Elbow by the eye
– Finish firm

Underhand:
– Ball on shoulder
– Drip of sweat
– 1, 2, punch

Queens of the Court
Team Drill

Number of Players: All

Player Positions: Three Lines on Baseline

Instructions

Players line up in three lines on the baseline while coach is across the net from the Queen side with a cart of volleyballs. First player in each line are the Queens (Q). As the Queens dip under the net to find the Royal Courtyard, the Princesses (P) step on to challenge them. The coach always tosses across the net to the Queen side. If either side attempts three hits by passing a controlled pass up to the setter's zone, the coach grants a life and that team gets a "do over." A life is a way to emphasize three hits volleyball. When a play ends, new Challengers (CH) come onto the floor and either the Queens remain (Queens won the point) or new Queens run under the net to take over (Princesses won the point). Whichever side lost the point always shags the volleyball and returns to their lines. For an uneven number of players encourage new partners.

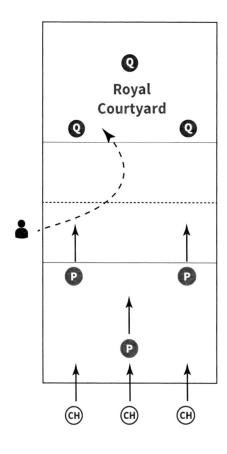

Cues

- Queens receive ball
- Call, "Free ball!" on coach's slap
- **Earn a life:** pass goes to setter zone
- **Queens win point:** Queens stay, Challengers step on
- **Princesses win point:** Queens off, Princesses move to Queen side, Challengers step on

Red, White, and Blue Hitting
Hitting Drill

Number of Players: All   **Player Positions:** Three Lines on Baseline

Instructions

This basic striking drill is about ball alignment on the hitting shoulder and learning to hit with an open hand. Players must ask for the ball by yelling, "Red, red, red!," "White, white, white!" or "Blue, blue, blue!" Once the coach hears them calling for the ball, the coach tosses a high toss. Players shuffle to get their shoulder lined up with the ball, point with their off-hand to the ball (track), and get into the trophy top pose. Stepping with the opposite foot and smacking the ball should be complete with a "firm finish," the statue pose at the end where the player is not falling off balance after contact.

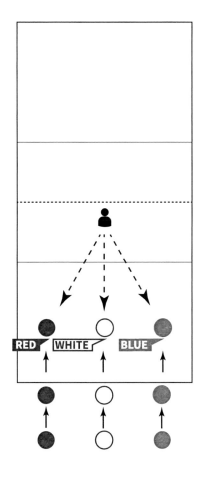

Cues

- Shoulder on ball
- High elbow
- Reach
- Trophy top
- Track and smack
- Finish firm

Baseline Throws
Serving, Hitting Drill

Number of Players: All

Player Positions: Baseline

Instructions

To help develop a fast striking arm, quick rotating hips, and a high elbow release or contact point, players throw from the baseline, over the net and into designated areas with various point values. Players are encouraged to throw with a higher than normal arm and the coach can make it a challenge for individual scores or a team personal best. Putting two teams against each other and allowing three throws each can make things more competitive and fun too.

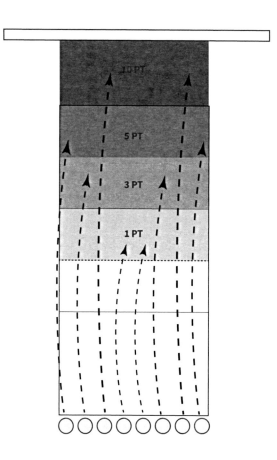

Cues

– Elbow starts up high
– Elbow by the eye
– Open and close hips
– Fast arm and fast hips
– Finish firm

Number of Players: Partners

Player Positions: Partners Across Net

Instructions

Players have a partner across the net. With a slap the tosser says, "It's up!" and tosses the ball over the net. The receiver shuffles to get their hips to the ball and catches with a long and strong platform. The ultimate goal is claiming the ball by calling "My ball, my ball!" before the ball gets over the net. Young players very new to the game believe you call the ball as it contacts the platform, so calling the ball before is usually a new challenge.

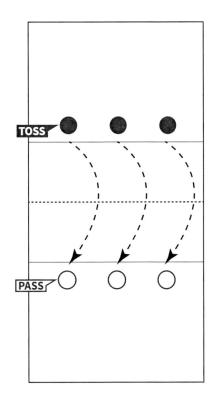

Cues

– Passers in ready stance
– Claim, "My Ball," before toss crosses the plane of the net
– Claim, don't blame!
– Catch the ball before it hits the ground
– Feet-feet freeze
– Hips to the ball
– **Goal:** early claim

Rotation Position Frogs
Lesson: Floor Position

Number of Players: All

Player Positions: Floor Positions

Instructions

With a 6 vs 6 look on the floor, players are down in a frog hopping position. Once floor positions are taught (right back, middle front, left front, etc.), players compete across the net with the other frog in their floor position. So as the coach yells out, "Left back," the two left back frogs pop up and ribbet! Whoever is faster, wins that round. Score can be kept but usually it's just fun to hop and laugh as they learn the floor positions. Remember to rotate every 4-8 times of yelling out the various positions, this will let the players rest their legs from the frog position.

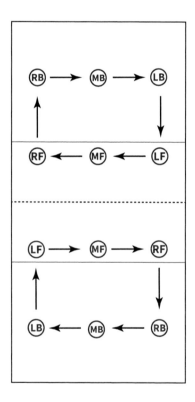

Cues

– Rotate clockwise

Floor Positions:
– RB: right back
– MB: middle back
– LB: left back
– LF: left front
– MF: middle front
– RF: right front

Number of Players: All   **Player Positions:** Half on Each Baseline

Instructions

On the coaches "Go," players race to serve two in-a-row. Once a player serves two in-a-row they yell out "One!" Every time a player successfully serves two in-a-row over, the team adds another number, "Two," "Three," until the team gets to ten.

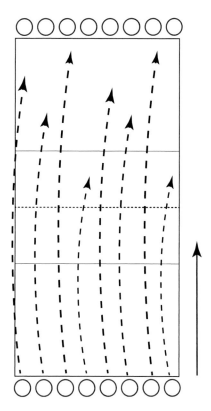

Cues

– 10 toes to target
– Players must communicate
– Lots of talking

Queen of the Throne
Passing Drill

Number of Players: Groups of 4 or 5   **Player Positions:** One Group on Each Side

Instructions

A chair is set out on the floor, close to the net where the Queen (Q) can sit on their throne! The Queen has a Peasant (P) working next to her. The Peasant is their royal tosser. The Peasant tosses to the 3 Princesses (PR), they are the passers who want to be the Queen. The sportsmanlike component to the challenge is that the Queen must try to catch a pass but they cannot come off their throne, so their bum must be on the throne at all times. Once a Princess's ball has been caught, they replace the old Queen so that there's a new queen. Every one or 2 minutes, the coach can yell out, "New Peasant!" (new tosser) and the challenge and fun continues. An extra player is the Joker (J) who shags and keeps a ball in the Peasant's hand.

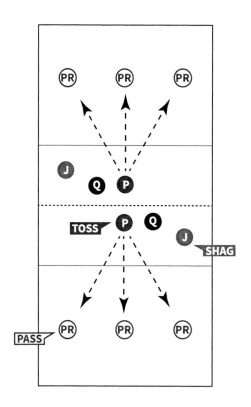

Cues

– The shagger keeps the drill going
– The Queen must try to catch the ball

Court Setup:

– Q: Queen tries to catch passes
– P: Peasant tosses the balls to the passers
– PR: Princesses try to pass the ball to the Queen
– J: Joker shags the ball

Number of Players: Partners

Player Positions: Net to Baseline

Instructions

Spacial awareness to the ball is our goal. Players learn to position their hips to the ball while distancing themselves from the volleyball. An open-close-open platform teaches players to move with their hands apart and place them together before contacting the ball. One partner, with their back on the net - a step or two in is fine, and the other partner a step or so in from the baseline allows partners to toss back and forth. The one bounce can get a little tougher as the drill moves along.

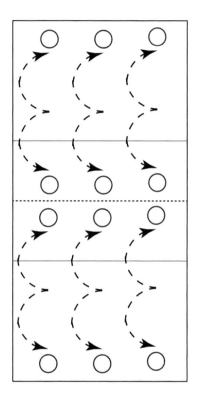

Cues

– Starts with a toss
– One bounce
– Distance from the ball
– Feet, feet, freeze
– Open-close-open platform

Volleyball Jog
Warm-up Drill

Number of Players: All

Player Positions: Around Court

Instructions

The players go for a light and easy jog around the floor - as a team! With a ball under their arm, players stop on coaches whistle and as they "rest" they perform a series of ball handling challenges such as popcorn, down balls, and self-sets. Once a challenge is over, players go another lap or two awaiting the whistle for their next task. This is a good ball handling activity.

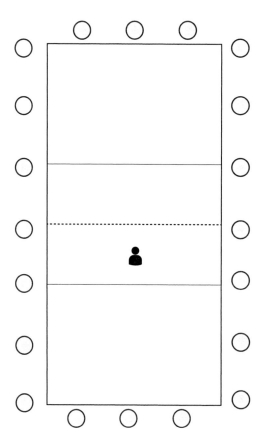

Cues

– Team jogs around the court
– Big and soft hands when setting
– Long and strong arms when passing

Challenges:
– Popcorn
– Self-sets
– Low passing catches
– Floor down balls

Shuffle, Shuffle, Freeze "Dance"
Passing Drill

Number of Players: All

Player Positions: Evenly Spaced

Instructions

Players are positioned in a group formation in lines, with plenty of room. Like a team dance, players follow the coaches lead and call out the footwork. Players move together in a rhythm going six to eight different directions. The coach can define the directions prior to beginning. Players must stay low and get through the six to eight spots and recover back to the middle each time. Remember coaches to face the net or have your back to the players so they can truly mirror your moves.

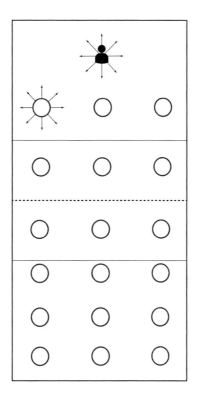

Cues

- "Dance" starts in ready stance on whistle
- Coach points the pattern and leads players in saying, "Feet, feet, freeze!" or "1, 2, freeze!"

REC+ Factor: Add a simulated movement of passing or setting at the completion of each footwork pattern.

Three Hits Goal
Hitting Drill

Number of Players: All

Player Positions: Three Hitting Lines

Instructions

Outside, middle, and right side hitters are lined up eager to jump and swing. The coach sets a goal for the team, for example, 10 good swings. From a coach's toss, players take a full approach, jump, and hit. Coach may also challenge the three hitters with asking for a particular hit: tip, off-speed, line shot, cross-court shot, deep corner, etc. When the individual hitter is successful with the coach's call, they add a point to the team goal.

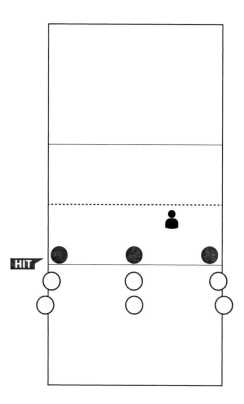

Cues

– Coach tosses to the hitters
– Player's echo coach's call

Work on commands for:
– Tips
– Off Speed
– Line
– Cut
– Cross Court

Year Four

Year Four is the perfect age for a real 6 vs 6 look! While never "scrimmaging," there are fun and effective lead-up games and challenges you will find in your curriculum to get the Year Four players excited. Add wall work and introduce "what to say and when to say it." For example, the setters says "I go, I go!" When it's not your ball you say, "Go-Go-Go" which in volleyball language means its not mine.

Players start learning how to move on the floor - 10 toes to the ball and never standing still. Short-court games are fun, challenging all players to collectively score points. While keeping score is appropriate, removing players or "elimination games" will quickly discourage at this age. One way to keep score while making sure it is not a big factor is insist on "modest celebration by everyone at the end of play.

Year 4

Practice Schedule
Year Four

	Page	Drill
Week 1	247	Lesson: Practice Management
	87	Early Bird Special
	88	Dynamic Warm-up
	89	Team Stretch
	90	Four Muscle Memory Throws
	246	Lesson: Passing
	250	Partner Passing
	246	Lesson: Lateral Footwork
	91	Rapid Fire Passing
	250	Wall Work: Underhand and Overhand Serving
	92	Perfect Ups
Week 2	87	Early Bird Special
	250	Partner Passing
	93	Juggling Patterns
	94	Wall Work Series
	242	VOLLEYBALL 10,000™
Week 3	87	Early Bird Special
	94	Wall Work Series
	251	Tennis Ball Wall Throws
	247	Lesson: Tracking, Shoulder and Ball Alignment
	95	Red, White, and Blue Hitting
	96	1-2 Passing Steps
	250	Serving for Correction
	97	Serve and Sprint
Week 4	87	Early Bird Special
	250	Jump Rope
	98	Toss, Pass, Target
	247	Lesson: Setting
	251	Wall Sets
	99	The "4" (Setting)
	100	Partner Setting
	101	Whistle Serves
	102	Serve One, Pass One
	103	Line Shuttle Drill

	Page	Drill
Week 5	87	Early Bird Special
	103	Line Shuttle Drill
	88	Dynamic Warm-up
	89	Team Stretch
	90	Four Muscle Memory Throws
	104	Baseline Throws
	105	Pass and Switch
	106	2-Step/4-Step Hitting
	107	Plyo Jumps and Hitting
	247	Lesson: Serve Receive
	108	3 LoBL Combo Touches
	109	10-in-30
	110	Jail Break
	111	Dead Fish
Week 6	87	Early Bird Special
	250	Jump Rope
	251	Wind Sprints
	112	12' Agility
	242	VOLLEYBALL 10,000™
	113	Queens of the Court
Week 7	87	Early Bird Special
	90	Four Muscle Memory Throws
	250	Partner Passing
	114	7-Up
	115	Serve Receive to Target
	116	Fill the Void
	117	3-Ball Speed Serving
	101	Whistle Serves
	118	Smart and Sweet Passes
Week 8		**Game Week**
	119	Pepper
	120	Free-Ball, Free-Ball, Free-Ball, Wash
	121	10x Hits, Tips, Dumps
	111	Dead Fish
	243	How Many Challenge
	122	Speed Ball

Year 4

Practice Schedule
Year Four

Early Bird Special
Warm-up Drill

Number of Players: All

Player Positions: Scattered

Instructions

The Early Bird Special (EBS) is all about hitting the ground running. Players get a ball immediately upon entering the gym and begin their EBS routine or the warm-up. Players stay engaged and repeat until the coach brings the full group together. The EBS should end the question, "what do we do?" as players arrive.

Example 1

1. Jog two laps
2. 20 floor down balls
3. 20 wall sets
4. 20 self-bumps
5. 10 wall serves

Example 2

1. 25 jumping Jills
2. 5 push ups
3. 20 wall serves
4. Pepper with a pal

Example 3

1. 50 popcorns
2. 50 self-sets
3. 50 down balls

Example 4

1. 20 net jumps
2. 30 partner passes and sets
3. 40 line runs

Cues

- Same or different challenges
- Serves as you warm-up
- Reviews and reinforces skills
- Immediate touches

Dynamic Warm-up
Warm-up Drill

Number of Players: All

Player Positions: Three Lines on Baseline

Instructions

Dynamic warm-up includes a series of stretches from high knees to bottom kicks. Players line up in three lines on the baseline and on the coach's whistle are brought out from their lines. Players can do the warm-up exercise to the net and back, with lots of high-fives and enthusiasm as they return to the line. Coach can emphasize players being **attentive** and **invested** in the details and remind the players to "lift toes," "drive the knee," "keep shoulders parallel with the wall," etc.

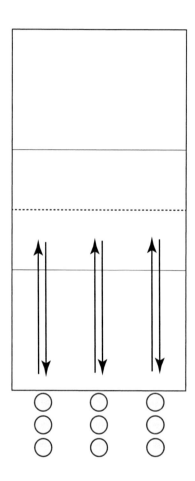

Suggested Exercises:

– High knee with a skip
– Bounds with a skip
– Butt kickers
– Grapevine
– Frankensteins
– Jogging, forwards and backwards

Number of Players: All   **Player Positions:** Lines

Instructions

The team is in lines, orderly and uniform. As the coach moves players through a series of static stretches the players stay involved and engaged by counting and holding the stretches. The coach yells out the **odd** numbers as the players count the **even** numbers. Players either clap two times or slap the floor two times after the 10 count and chant their team name!

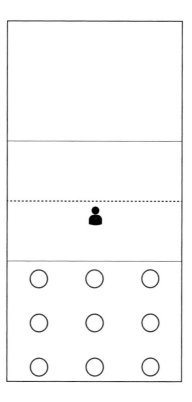

Suggested Stretches:

– RT over LT
– LT over RT
– Straddle
– Arm front and behind stretches
– Butterfly and hurdle stretch

Four Muscle Memory Throws
Warm-up Drill

Number of Players: Partners   **Player Positions:** Net to Baseline

Instructions

There are four muscle-memory throws:

1) Two Thumbs by the Thighs - players, positioned with a partner, throw for warm-up and also for developing essential movements in overhand serving, hitting, and hip rotation. Two Thumbs by the Thighs has partners bouncing the ball hard once to the floor - playing catch - back and forth.

2) Elbow by the Eye - players pause and adjust their throwing arm to get the throwing arm elbow "by the eye." As they throw with the opposite foot forward, the coach reminds players of the opening and closing of their hips. Players throw from high to low, meaning wrist snap at the release, aiming for the receiving partners knee pads.

3) Back to Your Partner - partners face away from their partner and step forward, with either foot to switch it up, arching the back and "throwing their chest to the ceiling" and holding their arms way up high pose.

4) Two Slaps and a Down Ball - two big open hand "slappy" sounds on the ball followed by a down ball to their partner. The ball bounces once. Remind players in this "throw" to not toss the ball but hit it out of their own hand or after a very small toss.

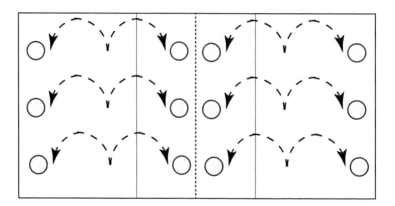

Cues

Throws:

1) Two Thumbs by the Thigh	Hard throws to the floor
2) Elbow by the Eye	Elbow starts high and leads
3) Back to Your Partner	Big and animated
4) Two Slaps and a Down Ball	Slaps with elbow lead

Number of Players: All

Player Positions: Net to Baseline

Instructions

The drill begins with a partner formation, one player with their back on the net and the partner on the baseline. On the coach's whistle, all tossers will slap the ball and say "It's up!" Passers claim and call the volleyball, "My ball, my ball," and "shovel" it up to the tosser. The tosser then becomes a setter, getting their feet set and receiving the ball on their setter's window. The target then yells out, "I go, I go!" as they see the ball coming into their hands. The target does not set it but simply catches the volleyball in their "setter's hands" making sure to shape the ball. Passers then rotate while the tossers stay put. Everyone should be ready and waiting for the next whistle.

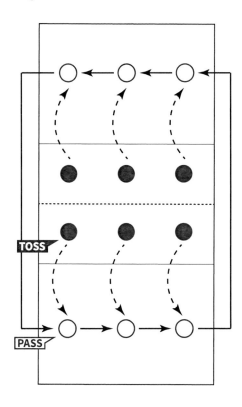 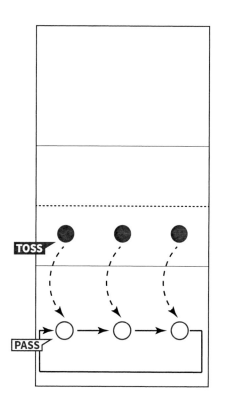

Cues

– Working together
– Players shuffle to the next tosser at the same time
– "One-Mississippi" hold after contact
– Shovel

Communicate:

– Toss: "It's up!"
– Pass: "My ball!"
– Target: "I go!"

Perfect Ups
Passing Drill

Number of Players: Partners

Player Positions: Net to Baseline

Instructions

Set players up in partner formation, one with their back on the net and the other near or around the baseline. The tossers immediately become the targets after they release the ball. The passer claims the ball and passes an antenna high (basketball rim-high) pass to the target. The target has a pivot foot and can only move as far as they can with that foot still in place. If the target can catch the ball with their pivot foot in the same place, the pass counts as a point. Passers **hold** the follow-through for a "one-Mississippi" count as the target works hard to catch the ball.

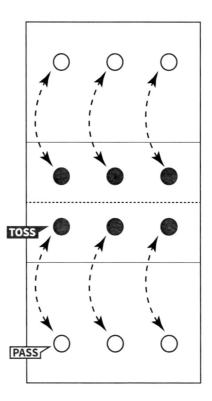

Cues

– Target has one foot "nailed" to floor
– "One-Mississippi" hold after contact
– A "perfect up" is antenna high pass

REC+ Factor: Coach puts time on the clock to see how many catches the partners can achieve. Another fun option is allowing a partners to see how many consecutive pass/catch points they can achieve.

Number of Players: All

Player Positions: Scattered

Instructions

Coach calls out a series of ball handling challenges. Coach may request a pattern of these challenges or a series. For example, coach yells out - "20 self-sets followed by 20 self bumps." The goal is to have ball control and numerous, fast touches.

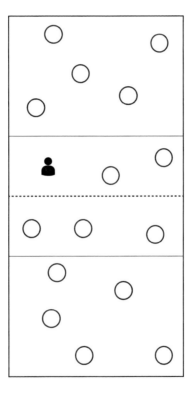

Cues

– Claim the ball
– Keep the ball in your own area

Challenges:

– Self bumps
– Self-sets
– Sand pokies
– etc.

Wall Work Series
Ball Control Drill

Number of Players: All   **Player Positions:** On Wall

Instructions

Wall work is for individual player development. Players find an area on the wall and move through a series of skills including: wall sets, wall down balls from a knee, wall down balls from standing, serving wall pins, serving wall deliveries or steady serving tosses, wall passing, and full wall serves , stepping off the wall 15-20 feet. This series can range from 30 seconds to 2 minutes per skill set.

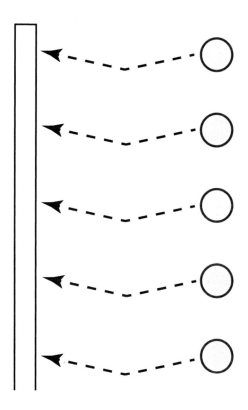

Drills

– Sets
– Down balls from knee
– Down balls standing
– Pins
– Tosses, shoulder on line
– Passes
– Serves

Number of Players: All   **Player Positions:** Three Lines on Baseline

Instructions

This basic striking drill is about ball alignment on the hitting shoulder and learning to hit with an open hand. Players must ask for the ball by yelling, "Red, red, red!," "White, white, white!" or "Blue, blue, blue!" Once the coach hears them calling for the ball, the coach tosses a high toss. Players shuffle to get their shoulder lined up with the ball, point with their off-hand to the ball (track), and get into the trophy top pose. Stepping with the opposite foot and smacking the ball should be complete with a "firm finish," the statue pose at the end where the player is not falling off balance after contact.

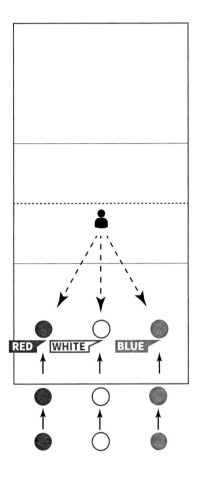

Cues

– Shoulder on ball
– High elbow
– Reach
– Trophy top
– Track and smack
– Finish firm

1-2 Passing Steps
Passing Drill

Number of Players: All

Player Positions: Two Lines

Instructions

This coach toss drill has two evenly divided lines. The drill will allow athletes to step, step or one, two step, to get to all tosses. The player's goal and the team goal should be to pass all balls back to the target using **only** two steps. Players model the skill footwork by saying, "1-2" or "Step, step" and eventually adding "1, 2, freeze, stick" before sticking their platform out for contact.

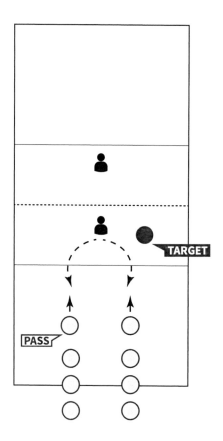

Cues

– Step, step, freeze
– A second coach can be added for an additional ball

Number of Players: Individual

Player Positions: Baseline

Instructions

Divide the team in half with each half on the serving baselines. Learning to "gain composure" after exertion, players serve and sprint to the opposite serving line. They reset their feet, take a deep breath, and start their routine. Once the player serves they practice calming down and being an effective server. The coach may put a certain amount of time on this challenge.

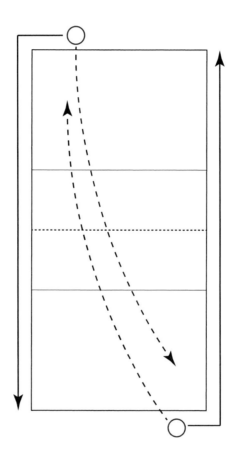

Cues

– Server's composure
– Exaggerate a deep breath to relax before serving

REC+ Factor: Conditioning drill, followed by composure

Toss, Pass, Target
Passing Drill

Number of Players: Groups of Three

Player Positions: Groups Across the Net or Groups on Same Side

Instructions

In their groups of three, players set up either across the net, for a longer toss, or on the same side, for a shorter toss. The tosser then slaps the ball and says, "It's up," before throwing the ball to the passer. The passer moves their feet to the ball and says, "My ball!" before passing the ball to the target. The target moves their feet to catch the ball in their "setter's window." The target then rolls the ball under the net back to the tosser. Have players rotate every 3 passes so that the tosser becomes the passer who becomes the target who is now the new tosser.

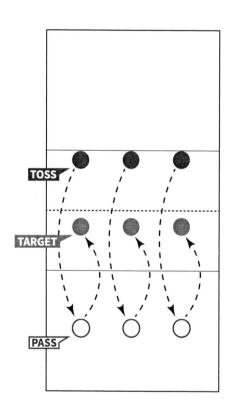 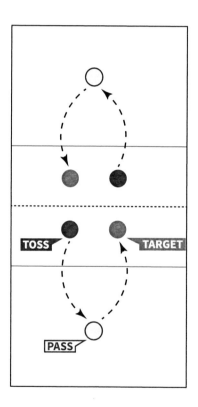

Cues

Communicate:
– Tosser: "It's up!"
– Passer: "My ball!"
– Target: "I go!"

REC+ Factor: Add a team goal or a time challenge.

Number of Players: All

Player Positions: Scattered

Instructions

Each player has a volleyball. From a self-toss, players self-set four consecutive sets. On the fourth set, players extend and set high. Players work to catch the ball with their "setter's hands" and "setter's feet." Players can "shape a panel" or find the 4-corners of a volleyball panel to begin the drill until they can maintain that hand positioning. Setter's feet has the right foot slightly forward with the left foot acting as a "kick-stand" like on their bike.

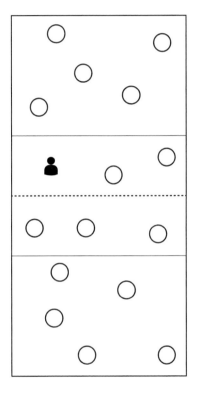

Cues

– Self set three and high set the fourth
– Count your sets: "One, two, three, four!"
– Feet, feet, freeze
– Shape the ball

Partner Setting
Setting Drill

Number of Players: Partners

Player Positions: Net to Baseline

Instructions

Players have a partner and are positioned on the floor across from one another. The tosser tosses from the baseline towards the net to the setter. The setter receives or catches the ball facing the tosser and then advances to turning their right shoulder on the net. Setters practice drawing theirs hands from the middle of their body up to the "setter's window." "Circle your belly-button" is a way to remind players how and where to rest their hands as they move to get to the ball. Setters can progress to a full set, in time.

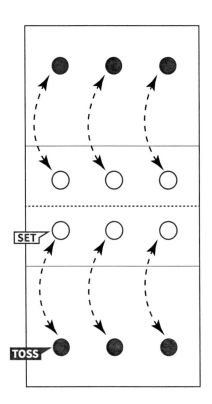

Cues

– Tossers need to toss high
– Setters move feet with 1-2 step
– Setters catch the first few then progress to full sets
– "Circle your belly button"

Number of Players: All

Player Positions: Starting at Net

Instructions

All players are serving at the same time in this drill. Players start with a ball at the net. The coach directs all players to hustle back to the baseline and begin their serving routine. Players pause and wait for the serving whistle and then all serve a few seconds thereafter. Building the official's whistle into the routine and teaching players to hustle back while limiting downtime is key to training for a strong muscle-memory serve. Players return to the net with their ball and prepare for several rounds of this drill.

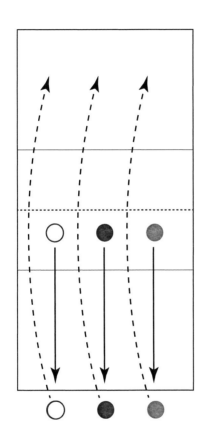
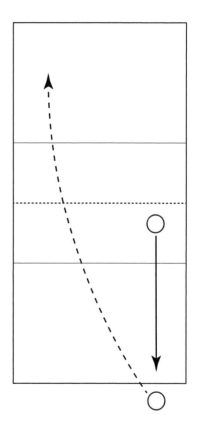

Cues

- Servers start at net with ball
- Hustle to baseline
- Listen and look for whistle
- Routine is key

Serve One, Pass One
Serving, Passing Drill

Number of Players: All

Player Positions: One Line or Two Lines

Instructions

This combo-drill allows for quick body positioning and game-like switching of skills. Players are in two lines facing the coach, who will toss from over the net. Players all have a ball in their hand. When it's the next players turn, that player will serve, then immediately step in to pass. Players should step into the floor quickly, widening their stance with each step. Hips then drop, drop, drop and hands do as well, preparing to pass. Players shag their **two** volleyballs, the serve and the pass, returning one to the cart and keeping the other for their next serve.

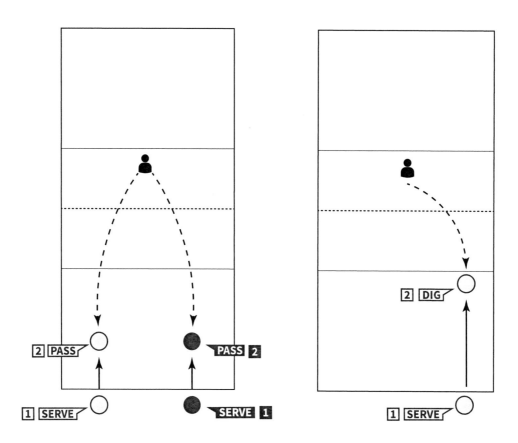

Cues

– Hustle onto the floor
– Get lower with each step
– Players can also dig the ball after their serve, the court on the right above

Number of Players: Groups of Five or Six   **Player Positions:** Two Lines Facing Each Other

Instructions

The coach divides the team into two even line facing one another with the first player in each line ready to pass or set. Starting with a toss across to the player in line, the first person passes or sets back to the line the ball started. After contact, players immediately run to the line they passed or set to. In other words, players pass or set and run to the back of the other line. This Shuttle Line keeps track of the number of consecutive touches. Coaches can challenge the team or lines to a personal team best or have two lines compete against one another. Also, adding time to the drill can challenge players to the number of no mess ups. A high pass or set allows for players to get in position for more success.

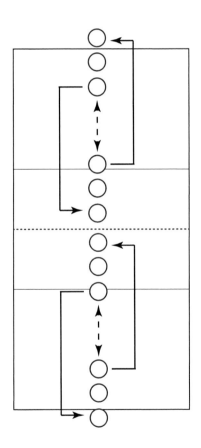
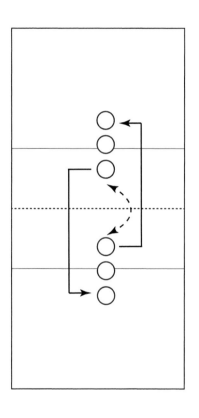

Cues

- Tosser chases their own toss to begin
- Passers follow their pass and join the back of the other line
- Feet first, then freeze
- "High buy times"
- Communication is key!

Baseline Throws
Serving, Hitting Drill

Number of Players: All

Player Positions: Baseline

Instructions

To help develop a fast striking arm, quick rotating hips, and a high elbow release or contact point, players throw from the baseline, over the net and into designated areas with various point values. Players are encouraged to throw with a higher than normal arm and the coach can make it a challenge for individual scores or a team personal best. Putting two teams against each other and allowing three throws each can make things more competitive and fun too.

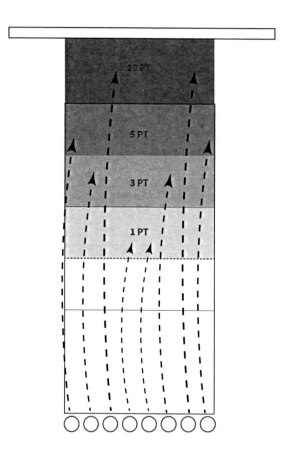

Cues

- Elbow starts up high
- Elbow by the eye
- Open and close hips
- Fast arm and fast hips
- Finish firm

Number of Players: Groups of Three

Player Positions: 2 Passers Near Baseline and Tosser at the Net

Instructions

The coach arranges players in groups of three with one tosser and two passers. The tosser has their back on the net. The tosser tosses the same course with each and every toss. The two passers are side by side. The first passer passes back to the tosser and both passers **quickly say**, "Switch, switch, switch!" The passer who passes the ball back to the tosser claims the volleyball by saying, "My ball, my ball!" and the non-passer **opens up** and says, "Go, go, go!" The coach calls out "New Tosser!" to rotate players. Keeping players in the drill for 30-45 seconds will place emphasis on being a low and ready passer. In this drill, **all players** are talking and communicating.

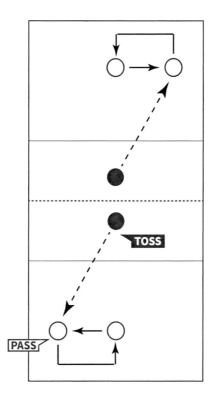

Cues

– Tosser tosses to the same spot every toss
– Passers switch with each pass
Players need to talk:
  – "Switch, switch, switch!"
  – "My ball!"
  – "Go, go, go!"

2 Step or 4 Step Drill
Hitting Drill

Number of Players: All   **Player Positions:** Hitting Lines

Instructions

In this drill each player will work without a ball. Players, as a group, will say the words "Step, close, up!" **Right-handed** players will have already taken their first step together, having the left foot forward a three step hitting approach would normally start with the right foot forward. A **left-handed** player would start with their right foot forward. Players rehearse step, close, up demonstrating their best "jumper's feet" and then, the coach adds the ball. From a coach toss, players work to line up their hitting shoulder with the ball and step, close, up to reach and spike the volleyball. The goal should be that all players work hard to contact the ball when in the air (feet off the floor) and work hard to keep the ball **out in front**. Coaches can back players up a step or two introducing the three step hitting approach or the 4-step hitting approach.

Cues

– Right-handed players: right, left, up
– Left-handed players: left, right, up
– Contact ball with their feet off the ground
– Shoulder on the ball
– Keep the ball in front

Plyo Jumps and Hitting
Hitting Drill

Number of Players: All

Player Positions: On Mats or Bleachers

Instructions

Set up as a station or a hitting footwork drill, players perform one at a time or as a team. Players, in a falling off the edge feeling, step, close at a slight angle turning 45 degrees to the right (for right handers) or left (for lefties). Players drop their hips and bottom back and load their legs to jump straight up. Players need to remember to throw their "elbows above their ears" for a big, aggressive jump. Players circle around and head back to the jumping line and wait for their next attempt. Consider a low step off height: 5-10" high.

Cues

- Step close and explode
- Use appropriate box height
- Can add other stations: jump rope, mini hurdles, etc.

3 LoBL Combo Touches
Ball Control Drill

Number of Players: All

Player Positions: Three Lines on Baseline

Instructions

3LoBL formation will have the first three athletes stepping into the floor. The coach communicates a series of touches or skill sets desired, for example: free ball, dig, track and smack. Players then, as a team demonstrate those skill sets in the order the coach called out. A combination of skills will determine how the coach will toss. Players are expected to call out the skill to communicate back to the coach the skill set they should be doing. Coach can emphasize some general cues throughout the drill like, frozen-feet, snap to draw setter's hands, shoulder to the ball when hitting.

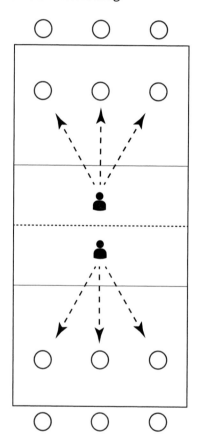

Cues

– Hip to the ball
– Fast toss
– Player call out their skill
– "Frozen feet" always priority

Coaches Commands:

– Pass
– Set
– Free ball
– Track and Smack

Number of Players: All

Player Positions: Baselines

Instructions

All players work hard to add a point to the team score by making their serve. The coach puts a certain amount of time on the clock and players work to successfully achieve the team goal that is set by the coach. For example, the coach may challenge their team to get 10 serves over in 30 seconds. Players are equally divided on each end and all volleyballs are out to use for quick serving. Players yell out "One," "Two," "Three," etc. counting **loudly** as each serve goes over the net.

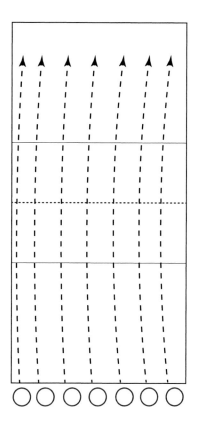

Cues

– Beat the clock
– Count loudly so everyone knows the number
– Timed drill with a goal

Jail Break
Serving Drill

Number of Players: All   **Player Positions:** Service Line

Instructions

All players serve from the Law Abiding Citizens side of the net. When a serve is missed the player who missed is "off to jail." There are two ways a player can get out of jail: coach yells "Jail break!" or a player claims a serve and catches it. If a player catches the volleyball from jail, they go back to the serving side and the player whose ball was caught goes to jail! This classic drill is always a team favorite.

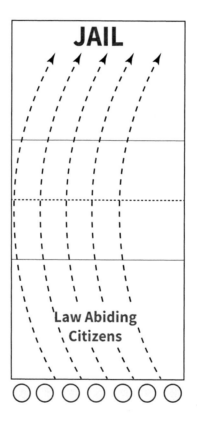

Cues

- Routine to punch
- **Good serve:** keep serving
- **Miss:** off to jail
- **Ticket out of jail:** catch a served ball
- **Serve is caught:** off to jail
- Coach may call "Jail break!" to free all

Number of Players: All

Player Positions: 2 Teams on Opposite Sides

Instructions

Coach divides the team into two even groups; the guppies and the goldfish! On the coach's whistle, all fish start serving. If a fish misses their serve, that server dips under the net to the other side's 10' line and sits criss-cross and is now a "dead fish." Live fish are trying to serve to their dead fish teammates because if a dead fish can catch a teammates' serve, they get to return to the live fish side. **All fish** keep serving to save and bring back their dead fish until all fish are dead. The side with the most live fish at the end of a certain time or the team with the most fish "alive," wins! If the team is playing without a clock/time, the winning fish are those with a minimum of **one** standing while the other team is all **dead fish**!

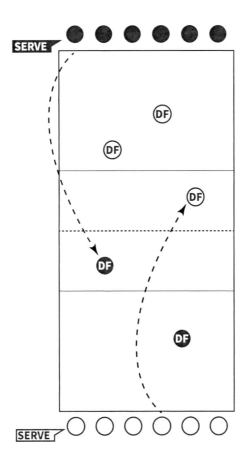

Cues

- Players keep serving till they miss
- Dead fish: player who has missed a serve
- Dead fish sit on the 10' line opposite of their team and try to catch a teammates serve
- If a dead fish catches a serve, they become a live fish again

12' Agility
Passing Drill

Number of Players: All   **Player Positions:** Net to Baseline

Instructions

Coach places an "X" on the floor (blue painters tape works well) and four marks are placed in a "t" shape from that "X." The distance from one mark to the "X" is six feet. One player starts at the "X" and the coach times their agility effort as they extend from one mark to the next, four touches total. The definition of agility will have players touching one mark, returning to the middle "X" and **switching directions**.

For example, a player starts at the "X" and goes to the **right**, touches the mark with their right hand and returns to the "X." Then, they head **forward** to the mark straight ahead, then back to the "X," then to the **left** mark and back to the "X," to complete the course the player must touch the last mark, **back**. To stop the clock, the player must go back to the "X" so that the player ends where they began. Players should work to compete against themselves first by improving their personal best time. **Footwork** should be "efficient" meaning as few steps as possible and emphasizing **reaching and extending** to touch the marks. Coach can add tosses at the marks for the player to pass.

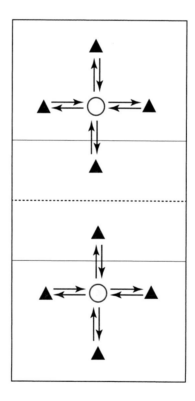

Cues

- Player starts in middle of the cones or marks, "X"
- Keep shoulder towards net
- Reach with foot and hand closest to mark
- Touch the marks counter-clockwise, or clockwise, never straight (right cone, "X," left cone)
- Low and extend

Number of Players: All

Player Positions: Three Lines on Baseline

Instructions

Players line up in three lines on the baseline while coach is across the net from the Queen side with a cart of volleyballs. First player in each line are the Queens (Q). As the Queens dip under the net to find the Royal Courtyard, the Princesses (P) step on to challenge them. The coach always tosses across the net to the Queen side. If either side attempts three hits by passing a controlled pass up to the setter's zone, the coach grants a life and that team gets a "do over." A life is a way to emphasize three hits volleyball. When a play ends, new Challengers (CH) come onto the floor and either the Queens remain (Queens won the point) or new Queens run under the net to take over (Princesses won the point). Whichever side lost the point always shags the volleyball and returns to their lines. For an uneven number of players encourage new partners.

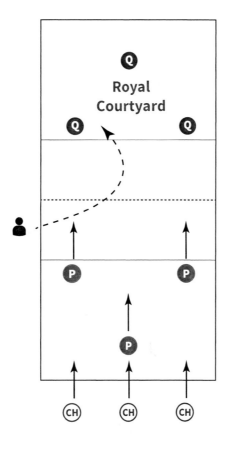

Cues

– Queens receive ball
– Call, "Free ball!" on coach's slap
– **Earn a life:** pass goes to setter zone
– **Queens win point:** Queens stay, Challengers step on
– **Princesses win point:** Queens off, Princesses move to Queen side, Challengers step on

7-Up
Passing, Setting, Hitting Drill

Number of Players: Groups of Three   **Player Positions:** Passer, Setter, and Hitter

Instructions

Coach divides the team into groups of three. The three players are: a tosser or setter, a passer and a hitter. The tosser has their back on the net facing the baseline and the passer is in the ready position, waiting to pass. The hitter, depending on whether they are right-handed or left, is positioned ready to down ball or hit the ball over. The drill begins with a toss, then a pass sends the ball back to the tosser and they set the ball out to the hitter. If the three players successfully accomplish all three skills, players **celebrate** with a "7-UP" loud, enthusiastic huddle up moment. If the three players get the three hits and the ball doesn't go over, the players huddle up for a not so enthusiastic "DIET 7-UP" call. The coach can rotate players every two to three minutes to make sure all players get to play at each position. Remember, **enthusiasm** and how to celebrate quickly and modestly is taught!

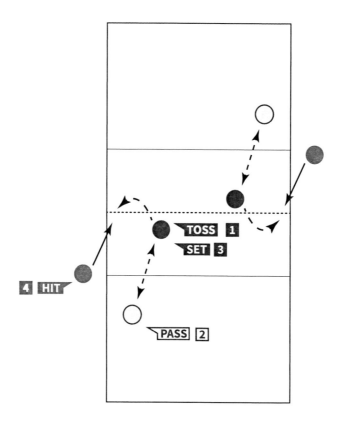

Cues

- 7-UP: A toss, pass, set, hit
- DIET 7-UP: A toss, pass, set, with the hit not going over
- Controlled contacts
- Communicate
- Celebrate

Number of Players: All

Player Positions: Three Lines on Baseline

Instructions

With three lines on the baseline the coach can either toss, underhand serve, or throw the volleyball over the net. Players receive the ball after claiming it, "baby it" up to the setter's zone. The coach sets a team goal of 10 to win and the challenge begins! Coach tosses, players rotate from passing to shagging, and the team yells out the number when there's a successful zone pass. As one player passes, the other two players should open up and say, "Go, go, go!"

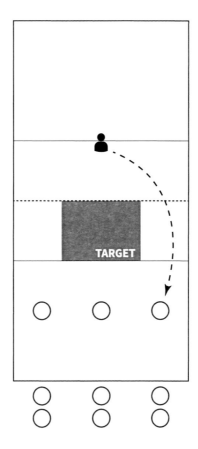

Cues

– Pass one and shag
– Accuracy is important
– Controlled touches
– Yell out score
– Smaller target can be extra bonus points

Fill the Void
Passing Drill

Number of Players: All   **Player Positions:** Three Lines on Both Baselines

Instructions

Half the team is on one side of the net in three lines on the baseline and the other half of players are mirroring that formation. The coach tosses from the same side of the net in this drill. From a toss, players focus on claiming the ball, receiving and passing it, while the nearest player "fills the void." Filling the void means two players pass as one player moves forward to the **setter's zone**. As the third hit goes over the net, the other side plays out the ball with the right back player also filling the void by running to the setter's zone. Once there's a dead ball or several attempts, players rotate, staying on their side of the net. Showing this in slow-motion may help players understand passing to a **zone** and not each other/not players.

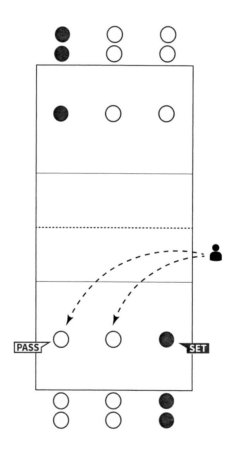

Cues

– Play out the ball
– Right back is the setter
– **Goal:** Always fill the zone

Number of Players: Individual   **Player Positions:** With a Line of Three Balls

Instructions

Three balls are placed on the floor. One at the 10' line with the player, one at the halfway point on the same side of the net, and one on the baseline. The server moves from ball to ball starting at the closest one to the net. Servers serve one ball and quickly go to the next and then to the third ball. The goal is for players to **not over think** but just pick up the ball and serve, serve, serve. Players stay true to their form and trust their skills. Their routine rehearsal is important and should look the same with every serve. Players should set the goal of making all three.

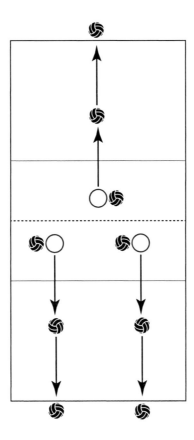

Cues

– Balls on 10', mid-court, and baseline
– Quick serves
– Use the same form for each distance
– Get feet set and do serving routine

Smart and Sweet Passes
Passing Drill

Number of Players: All

Player Positions: 3 Lines with Servers

Instructions

Players will love this challenge, because there's candy involved! All players decorate a paper lunch sack by drawing and coloring their name and some cool volleyball art! Players are positioned 3 across and with 3 on the floor at a time. The coach begins serving, tossing or throwing serves over the net and the passers "baby" the ball up to the defined setter's zone. When a player passes successfully to the setter's zone, they may go grab a candy and drop it in their Smart Passes paper bag. Players rotate after they shag their ball and hustle back to a line. Coaches may announce a **one minute bonus round** where a good pass is worth double the candy! To make sure every player receives at least one piece of candy, you may do candy for hustling, candy for communication, or candy for knowing the answer to a volleyball question.

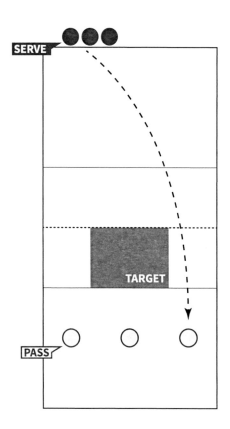

Cues

– Candy for a pass to the target
– Feet, feet, freeze
– "Stick the platform"
– "One-Mississippi" hold

REC+ Factor: Pick up the intensity level of your serves and make them tougher to receive.

Number of Players: Partners

Player Positions: Net to Baseline

Instructions

Players are partnered up factoring in skill level. Partners pepper using the cue words: **toss, pass, set, down ball, dig**. When players perform all five skills in-a-row, from the toss to the dig, the players yell out the **pepper** they accomplished or earned. For example, partners just peppered so the first time they accomplish this they yell out "Bell pepper," the second successful round they yell out, "Banana pepper," etc. Once a couple pairs get to the ghost pepper, the coach can throw out a **Carolina Reaper Pepper** challenge, three in-a-row non-stop peppers. Players are reminded to extend on their set then recover low to dig and to always recover back to the general area after each touch.

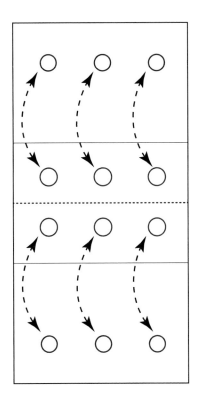

Peppers

– One pepper: Bell
– Two peppers: Banana
– Three peppers: Jalapeño
– Four peppers: Habanero
– Five peppers: Ghost

Free Ball, Free Ball, Free Ball, Wash
Team Drill

Number of Players: All   **Player Positions:** Three Lines on Baseline

Instructions

Players line up in three lines on the baseline. Players are sent out to the court in a "wash" drill formation, playing 6 vs 6, or 3 vs 3 if there are not enough players. The coach tosses over the net to the side **opposite** from the three lines. From the toss the players play volleyball. After three free ball tosses from the coach, players all yell "Wash!" and players rotate up the floor. When players wash off the court they shag their three volleyballs and return to their lines. An uneven number works fine, the players file in as they come back around the floor to the 3LoBL. The team goal and goal for every player should be to be "always talking and always moving."

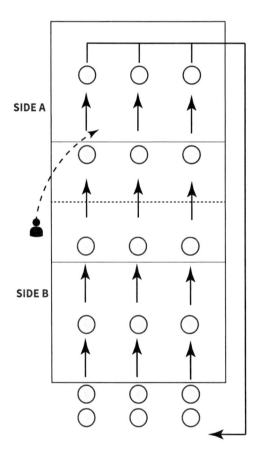

Cues

– Three free ball tosses form the coach
– After three free balls have been played out, wash
– 6 vs 6 or 3 vs 3
– Always talking
– Always moving

Number of Players: All

Player Positions: Three Lines on Baseline

Instructions

Three lines on the baseline allows three hitters to step up and get ready to swing! Players hit one and dip under the net to shag after the contact. A team goal of 10 tips, 10 hits, and 10 shoot sets **add up** to 30 successful hits. The goal could be as simple as 10 total of one of the front row hits the coach calls out. Footwork coaching cues include a first step "raise the roof" a step-close which is "mountain skier" to a big jump and a "trophy top" reach.

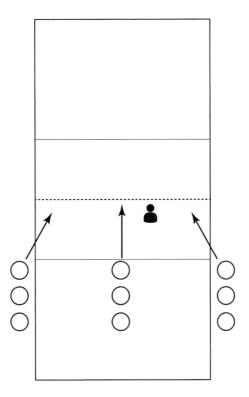

Cues

– Emphasis on strong step-close

Footwork Cues:
– Raise the roof
– Mountain skier
– Trophy top

REC+ Factor: The coach may call out the specific hits

Speed Ball
Team Drill

Number of Players: Groups of Three or Four

Player Positions: Three or Four Lines on Baseline

Instructions

Lines on the baseline will organize players for either 3 vs 3 play or 4 vs 4 play. Every touch is a point. The coach puts the ball in play with a free ball and players earn up to 3 points on one side, but the ball could be returned for additional points. Players play the free ball toss until it's defined dead and the players wash. The free ball toss always goes to side A. Players keep the **same teammates**.

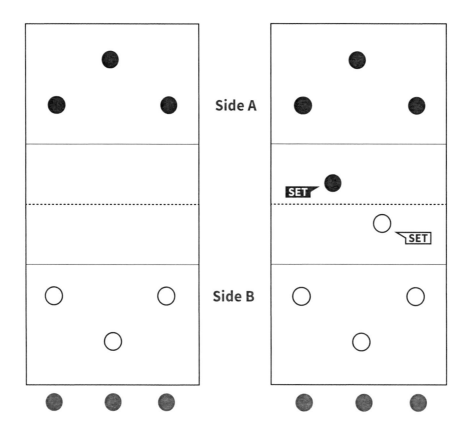

Cues

– 4 vs 4 wash
– Every touch is a point
– A touch is any contact with effort

REC+ Factor: a true three hits play where the hit goes over the net can result in a bonus 2 points, so the team would get 5 points instead of 3. The winning team does three push-ups while the non-winning team does 5 push-ups. The coach can reshuffle players and play another round!

Over the Net Pepper
Ball Control Drill

Number of Players: Partners

Player Positions: Partners Across the Net

Instructions

This is self pepper! Partners are positioned across the net from one another. From a toss over the net the receiving partner passes, sets, and hits the ball back over to their partner. The tosser may catch the ball and start again or can try to also self-pepper. This drill can also be done on one side of the net. Players try to control movements and communicate the skills while keeping the ball going back and forth.

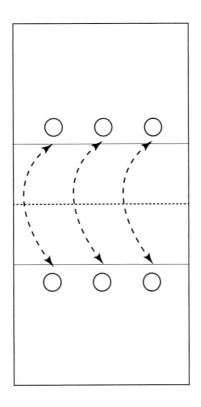

Cues

- Starts with a good toss
- Partner must pass, set, and hit
- Controlled movements
- Communicate and talk

Mock Serving
Serving Drill

Number of Players: Partners

Player Positions: Partners Across Net

Instructions

Partners are across the net from one another starting at the 10' line. The receiving partner is a big target with hands up, ready to catch. Serving partner is focused on the details of serving as coach places emphasis and reminders on the toss, the ball alignment, the punch, etc. Players are asked to take one step back after a few minutes of serving.

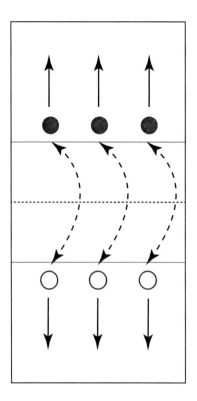

Cues

Overhand:
– Toss, step, punch
– Elbow by the eye
– Finish firm

Underhand:
– Ball on shoulder
– Drip of sweat
– 1, 2, punch

Number of Players: All

Player Positions: Three Lines on Baseline

Instructions

Players are positioned in three lines on the baseline. The coach is on the same side of the players with the cart and volleyballs. With six players on the floor, the coach slaps the ball and says "It's up!" The coach's toss is the first hit, meaning the side of six only has two more contacts to get the ball over the net. The coach's toss is a "bad pass" and the next two hits are the "good save." This drill is a real game-like drill. It helps prepare the team for a less-than-great first pass. The second hit or first save should be brought back to the middle of the floor so the team can call out the third hit. The team must survive the bad pass and make something good come out of things. The three diggers on the other side of the net help shag and may play it out, if time permits. Players rotate on the wash call by the coach. Passers move up to the front row, the front row dips under the net and become the new diggers, the old diggers shag any balls that are out then hop back in line.

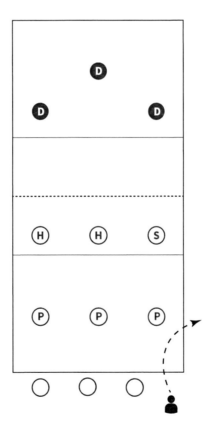

Cues

– 6 vs 3 wash drill
– Coach's toss is the first contact
– The team of six has two more contacts to get the ball over the net
– Run and hustle to ball with "runner's arms"

Reds and Outsides Hitting
Hitting Drill

Number of Players: All

Player Positions: 2 Hitting Lines

Instructions

The team is divided into two equal hitting lines. The outside attackers (O) are lined up near the 10' line outside of the court. Positioned not far behind them and inside the floor are the back row attackers (R). The outside hitters are calling out "4, 4, 4!" The back row attackers are calling out "Red, red, red!" The name of these attacking positions vary from state to state, by program, and by coach. Hitters hit the outside or the back row attack and dip under the net to shag and return to the hitting lines.

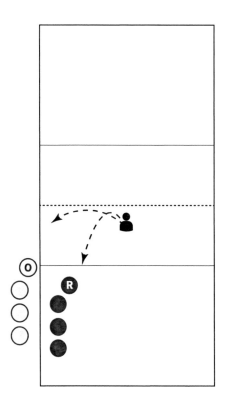

Cues

- Hitters switch lines
- Call for sets
- Outsides: "4,4, 4!"
- Back row: "Red, red, red!"
- Adjust footwork and angle of approach

Year Five

Year Five players are excited to learn and play "like the older kids" While making sure partnering up becomes the concern of the coach, players may begin sizing themselves up in terms of skill development and general skill benchmarks. This sensitive time is critically important when teaching how to encourage one another. Modeling, practicing, and recognizing strong sportsmanlike behavior will be helpful.

Coaches can add more combo drills where, for example, a dig may directly follow a serve and where a hit may follow a pass. An emphasis should be placed on three hits volleyball. Big celebrations should be taught and adding expectations of high energy to the floor may instill a habit of talking, moving, and encouraging. Simple player roles are identified by the coach and defining each role will help in the three hits goal. An example of this is, "When in right front, you're the setter. The setter works to get all second hits." Or asking players to identify their role, "I'm a passer.," "I'm a setter.," etc.

Year 5

Practice Schedule
Year Five

	Page	Drill
Week 4	131	Early Bird Special
	250	Jump Rope
	153	Jump Training x6
	154	Red, White, and Blue Hitting
	155	Alligator Attacks
	156	Pretzel
	157	Step and Stick
	158	Serve and Sprint
	159	Free Ball, Free Ball, Free Ball, Attack
Week 5	131	Early Bird Special
	160	Volleyball Jog
	161	Graduation Down Ball
	162	8 in 8
	163	Exert and Score
	164	Dig One, Serve One
	165	Rapid Fire Passing
	166	Set the Setter
	167	10 to Win
	168	Won It, Lost It, Tied It
Week 6	131	Early Bird Special
	169	Pepper
	241	Personal Best Score Card (Year 4-6)
	251	Wall Work
	136	Juggling Patterns
	170	Line Shuttle Drill
	171	Three Short, Three Deep
	172	Hit and Exit
	173	Dig to Hit
Week 7		**Game Week**
	132	Dynamic Warm-up
	133	Team Stretch
	174	Jail Break
	175	Spider Web
	176	Free Ball, Free Ball, Free Ball, Wash
	177	Jump Train

Practice Schedule
Year Five

Number of Players: All

Player Positions: Scattered

Instructions

The Early Bird Special (EBS) is all about hitting the ground running. Players get a ball immediately upon entering the gym and begin their EBS routine or the warm-up. Players stay engaged and repeat until the coach brings the full group together. The EBS should end the question, "what do we do?" as players arrive.

Example 1

1. Jog two laps
2. 20 floor down balls
3. 20 wall sets
4. 20 self-bumps
5. 10 wall serves

Example 2

1. 25 jumping Jills
2. 5 push ups
3. 20 wall serves
4. Pepper with a pal

Example 3

1. 50 popcorns
2. 50 self-sets
3. 50 down balls

Example 4

1. 20 net jumps
2. 30 partner passes and sets
3. 40 line runs

Cues

– Same or different challenges
– Serves as you warm-up
– Reviews and reinforces skills
– Immediate touches

Dynamic Warm-up
Warm-up Drill

Number of Players: All   **Player Positions:** Three Lines on Baseline

Instructions

Dynamic warm-up includes a series of stretches from high knees to bottom kicks. Players line up in three lines on the baseline and on the coach's whistle are brought out from their lines. Players can do the warm-up exercise to the net and back, with lots of high-fives and enthusiasm as they return to the line. Coach can emphasize players being **attentive** and **invested** in the details and remind the players to "lift toes," "drive the knee," "keep shoulders parallel with the wall," etc.

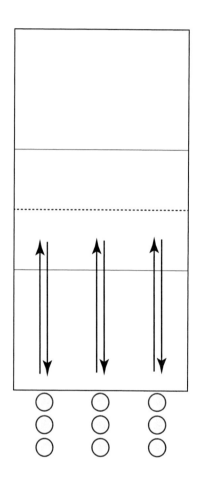

Suggested Exercises:

– High knee with a skip
– Bounds with a skip
– Butt kickers
– Grapevine
– Frankensteins
– Jogging, forwards and backwards

Number of Players: All

Player Positions: Lines

Instructions

The team is in lines, orderly and uniform. As the coach moves players through a series of static stretches the players stay involved and engaged by counting and holding the stretches. The coach yells out the **odd** numbers as the players count the **even** numbers. Players either clap two times or slap the floor two times after the 10 count and chant their team name!

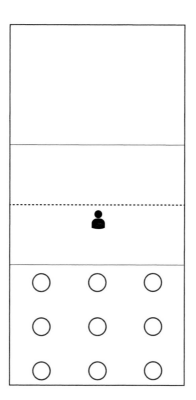

Suggested Stretches:

– RT over LT
– LT over RT
– Straddle
– Arm front and behind stretches
– Butterfly and hurdle stretch

Four Muscle Memory Throws
Warm-up Drill

Number of Players: Partners

Player Positions: Net to Baseline

Instructions

There are four muscle-memory throws:

1) Two Thumbs by the Thighs - players, positioned with a partner, throw for warm-up and also for developing essential movements in overhand serving, hitting, and hip rotation. Two Thumbs by the Thighs has partners bouncing the ball hard once to the floor - playing catch - back and forth.

2) Elbow by the Eye - players pause and adjust their throwing arm to get the throwing arm elbow "by the eye." As they throw with the opposite foot forward, the coach reminds players of the opening and closing of their hips. Players throw from high to low, meaning wrist snap at the release, aiming for the receiving partners knee pads.

3) Back to Your Partner - partners face away from their partner and step forward, with either foot to switch it up, arching the back and "throwing their chest to the ceiling" and holding their arms way up high pose.

4) Two Slaps and a Down Ball - two big open hand "slappy" sounds on the ball followed by a down ball to their partner. The ball bounces once. Remind players in this "throw" to not toss the ball but hit it out of their own hand or after a very small toss.

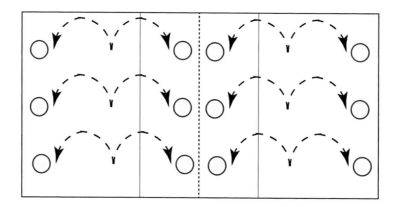

Cues

Throws:

1) Two Thumbs by the Thigh	Hard throws to the floor
2) Elbow by the Eye	Elbow starts high and leads
3) Back to Your Partner	Big and animated
4) Two Slaps and a Down Ball	Slaps with elbow lead

Number of Players: All

Player Positions: Circles

Instructions

Players learn to individually control the ball by "popping," passing to themselves. The quick punch or pop right before contact is the goal. Players have fun alternating their popcorn or by seeing how many consecutive popcorn contacts they can complete. Coaches can add to the challenge by adding the one-two-cross, meaning two contacts on one arm and pop it over to two contacts on the other. Remind players to have their hips behind their heels in an active, athletic stance. Also, do not reach for the ball but shuffle over with active feet.

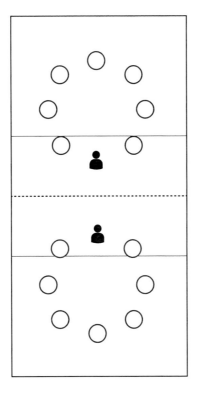

Cues

– Active feet
– Athletic stance
– Be vocal, count out loud

Juggling Patterns
Ball Control Drill

Number of Players: All　　　　　　　　　　　**Player Positions:** Scattered

Instructions

Coach calls out a series of ball handling challenges. Coach may request a pattern of these challenges or a series. For example, coach yells out - "20 self-sets followed by 20 self bumps." The goal is to have ball control and numerous, fast touches.

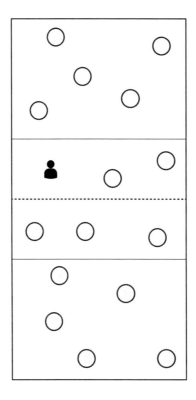

Cues

– Claim the ball
– Keep the ball in your own area

Challenges:
– Self bumps
– Self-sets
– Sand pokies
– Floor down balls

Belly Up Passing
Passing Drill

Number of Players: All

Player Positions: Three Lines on Baseline

Instructions

Players line up in three lines on the baseline and step onto the floor and go right to their bellies! On the coach's slap of the ball, all three players pop up and the coach tosses to one. The one who is passing the ball claims the ball and passes it to the setter's zone while the other two passers yell "Go, go, go!" Players return to their belly and get ready to pop up and play again. Players are encouraged to pop up **low** and in the "ready position." The coach makes sure they have tossed to every player!

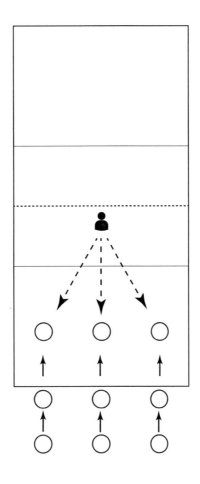

Cues

– Players start on their bellies
– Passer: "My ball!"
– Others: "Go, go, go!"
– Players should pop up low instead of popping up high and then getting low

Be the Board
Passing Lesson

Number of Players: All　　　　　　**Player Positions:** Circled Around Coach

Instructions

This is a coach demonstration of how to not swing when passing the volleyball. Using a 1ft by 4ft board that is 1" thick, the coach shows how the board is just like a "long and strong" platform. There's a high, rainbow toss and a no-swinging pass back to the target. Coach emphasizes a wide base with frozen feet, hips to the ball, and the lifting of legs to "shovel" the ball back to the target.

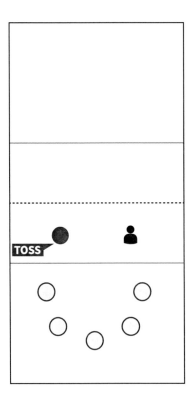

Cues

– Coach sitting in a chair
– Using board to pass back to target
– 1-2 step
– Frozen feet
– "Shovel" back to target

Number of Players: Groups of Three

Player Positions: Two Passers Near Baseline and Tosser at the Net

Instructions

The coach arranges players in groups of three with one tosser and two passers. The tosser has their back on the net. The tosser tosses the same course with each and every toss. The two passers are side by side. The first passer passes back to the tosser and both passers **quickly say**, "Switch, switch, switch!" The passer who passes the ball back to the tosser claims the volleyball by saying, "My ball, my ball!" and the non-passer **opens up** and says, "Go, go, go!" The coach calls out new tosser to rotate players. Keeping players in the drill for 30-45 seconds will place emphasis on being a low and ready passer. In this drill, **all players** are talking and communicating.

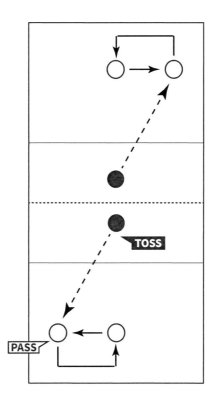

Cues

– Tosser tosses to the same spot every toss
– Passers switch with each pass

Players need to talk:
– "Switch, switch, switch!"
– "My ball!"
– "Go, go, go!"

Coach Toss Serving
Serving Drill

Number of Players: All

Player Positions: Multiple Lines

Instructions

To eliminate the one thing that many times gets in the way of the overhand serve, the toss, let's have the coach tossing for the players. Players form two lines or one line per coach. The coach positions the volleyball out in front of the server's hitting shoulder. The player has their striking hand on top of the ball, relaxed. When the coach says, "Pull," the player pulls the hand back over their head and shoulder area with their 4 fingertips facing the ceiling. The player does not have their off hand or tossing hand anywhere near the ball. The player serves the toss. The cue after the player pulls their striking hand from the ball is, "Step, punch!" The front foot slightly steps (more of a weight transfer) and with the open hand they accelerate or punch the ball. This allows the player to focus on torque or twisting of their hips, shoulder rotation, and a "finish firm" finale. Remind servers to **drag** their back toe to the front heel as this slows the hips down for a much more controlled contact. Players shag their ball and return to the serving lines.

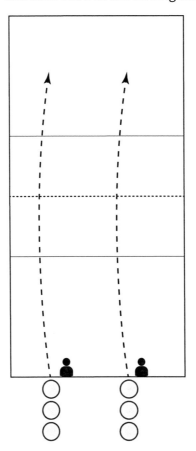

Cues

– Step and punch
– Finish firm

Coach says:

– "Pull!" - player takes hand off the ball
– "Toss!" - throw the ball up in front of the hitting shoulder
– "Step, punch!" - instruct the player to put their body into the serve

www.theartofcoachingvolleyball.com

Number of Players: All   **Player Positions:** Gathered Around Coach

Instructions

As a group, the coach stands in front of the players, eventually with their back to the players for the purpose of being able to mirror movements. Players repeat the rhythm of the overhand serve. The coach says the step out loud and shows the step, then the players repeat. The rhythm includes the chant of the serving steps: 10 toes to the target, two dribbles, step back, cool spin, ball in front of the hitting shoulder, **toss-step-punch**. The players want to finish firm with a sense of control and upright posture in their follow through. Players may hold each position for a few seconds in the beginning so that the coach can tweak the details of their serving performance.

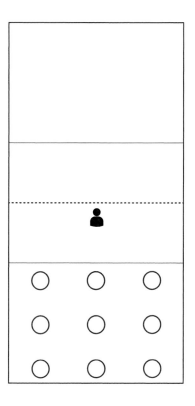

Cues

Coach repeats rhythm as players follow commands:
– 10 toes to target
– Two dribbles
– Step back with a cool spin
– Ball in front of the hitting shoulder
– Toss, step, punch
– Finish firm

7-Up
Passing, Setting, Hitting Drill

Number of Players: Groups of Three   **Player Positions:** Passer, Setter, and Hitter

Instructions

Coach divides the team into groups of three. The three players are: a tossser or setter, a passer and a hitter. The tosser has their back on the net facing the baseline and the passer is in the ready position, waiting to pass. The hitter, depending on whether they are right-handed or left, is positioned ready to down ball or hit the ball over. The drill begins with a toss, then a pass sends the ball back to the tosser and they set the ball out to the hitter. If the three players successfully accomplishes all three skills, players **celebrate** with a "7-UP" loud, enthusiastic huddle up moment. If the three players get the three hits and the ball doesn't go over , the players huddle up for a not so enthusiastic "DIET 7-UP" call. The coach can rotate players every two to three minutes to make sure all players get to play at each position. Remember, **enthusiasm** and how to celebrate quickly and modestly is taught!

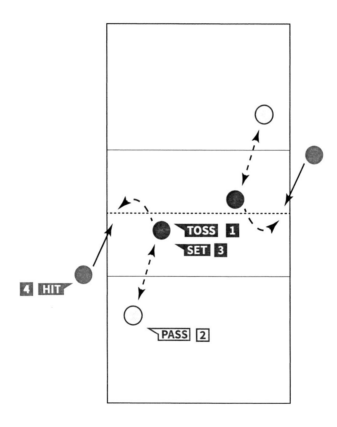

Cues

– 7-UP: A toss, pass, set, hit
– DIET 7-UP: A toss, pass, set, with the hit not going over
– Controlled contacts
– Communicate
– Celebrate

Number of Players: Individual

Player Positions: Net to Baseline

Instructions

Coach places an "X" on the floor (blue painters tape works well) and four marks are placed in a "t" shape from that "X." The distance from one mark to the "X" is six feet. One player starts at the "X" and the coach times their agility effort as they extend from one mark to the next, four touches total. The definition of agility will have players touching one mark, returning the the middle "X" and s**witching directions**.

For example, a player starts at the "X" and goes to the **right**, touches the mark with their right hand and returns to the "X." Then, they head **forward** to the mark, then **left**, last, to complete the course the player must touch the last mark, **back**. To stop the clock, the player must go back to the "X" so that the player ends where they began. Players should work to compete against themselves first by improving their personal best time. **Footwork** should be "efficient" meaning as few steps as possible and emphasizing **reaching and extending** to touch the marks. Coach can add tosses at the marks for the player to pass.

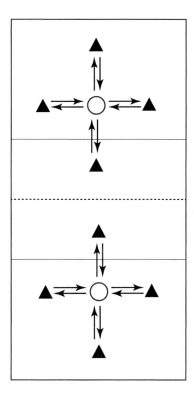

Cues

– Player starts in middle of the cones or marks, "X"
– Keep shoulder towards net
– Reach with foot and hand closest to mark
– Touch the marks counter-clockwise, or clockwise, never straight, ex: right cone, "X," left cone
– Low and extend

Baseline Throws
Serving, Hitting Drill

Number of Players: All

Player Positions: Baseline

Instructions

To help develop a fast striking arm, quick rotating hips, and a high elbow release or contact point, players throw from the baseline, over the net and into into designated areas with various point values. Players are encouraged to throw with a higher than normal arm and the coach can make it a challenge for individual scores or a team personal best. Putting two teams against each other and allowing three throws each can make things more competitive and fun too.

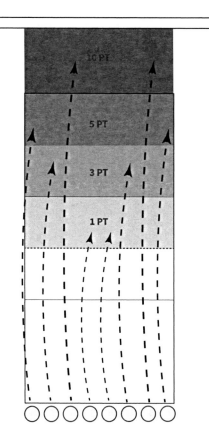

Cues

– Elbow starts up high
– Elbow by the eye
– Open and close hips
– Fast arm and fast hips
– Finish firm

Number of Players: All   **Player Positions:** Three Lines on Baseline

Instructions

3LoBL formation will have the first three athletes stepping into the floor. The coach communicates a series of touches or skill sets desired, for example: free ball, dig, track and smack. Players then, as a team demonstrate those skill sets in the order the coach called out. A combination of skills will determine how the coach will toss. Players are expected to call out the skill to communicate back to the coach the skill set they should be doing. Coach can emphasize some general cues throughout the drill like, frozen-feet, snap to draw setter's hands, shoulder to the ball when hitting.

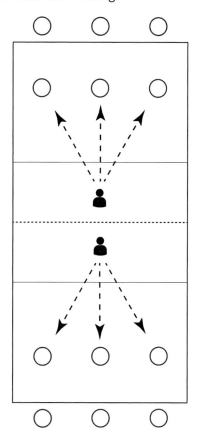

Cues

- Hip to the ball
- Fast toss
- Player call out their skill
- "Frozen feet" always priority

Coaches Commands:

- Pass
- Set
- Free ball
- Track and Smack

Butterfly
Team Drill

Number of Players: Groups of Five to Seven

Player Positions: Across the Net

Instructions

This drill has five to seven positions filled on half the floor that create a "modified" butterfly drill. When done on both halves, it takes the look of butterfly wings. The coach or tosser (T) is positioned 5-15 feet behind the 10' line. They toss to the setter (S). The setter can self-set a couple of times to gain control or a more advanced setter can simply set out to the outside hitter (H). The hitter hits as the blocker (B) goes up to block and the digger (D) is deeper in defense working to dig or get the touch. Hitters are encouraged to hit at the digger. The digger can either turn and shag that ball, or the coach can add a shagger to go get that ball, while all other players rotate up a position. Players must learn to follow the pattern of the ball to know where to rotate. With the drill occupying both sides of the floor it does best when it is set up opposite or facing one another again, forming that butterfly appearance.

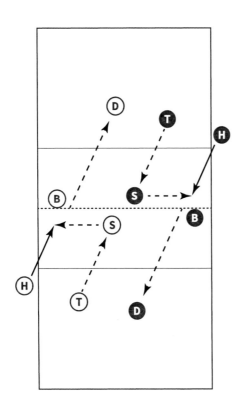 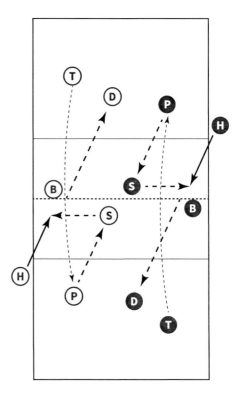

Cues

– Communicate
– Anticipate
– Alignment
– Feet first
– Tosser to Setter to Hitter to Blocker to Digger (to Shagger) to Tosser
– Tosser to Passer to Setter to Hitter to Blocker to Digger (to Shagger) to Tosser

Number of Players: All

Player Positions: 6 vs 6 Formation

Instructions

The transition fluidity drill is a walk-through type of drill that calls for players to use their imagination. Players will have specific places to rotate or move to as the coaches (two coaches needed) explain offense to hitter coverage to defense. The players are expected to repeat the transition they are in three times. Players say, "ready-ready" or "feet-feet" as they adjust to receive an imaginary free ball or "cover-cover" as they circle in to cover the hitter, or "down-down-down" to adjust and prepare on defense. The coach carries the ball around, lifting it and showing what situation is happening. Move in slow motion around the floor teaching the basic adjustments in transitioning. The coaches may begin tossing the ball to add a little speed and game-like movement to the transitions, but they players will only catch the volleyballs. Remember, players are expected to talk and communicate with every transition. The drill should look fluid-like in time.

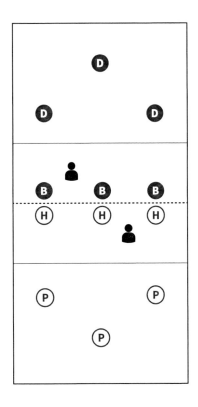

Cues

Players call out:
- Defense: "Down, down, down!"
- Coverage:" Cover, cover!"
- Offense: "Feet, feet!"

In-a-Nutshell Offense
Team Offense Lesson

Number of Players: All

Player Positions: 6 vs 6 Formation

Instructions

Players will learn the two primary serve-receive formations, the "W" and the "Cup." The coach will show how players come out of basic defense (three on front line, three on back line) to get into serve receive. Players will hear terms or cue phrases like, "push the setter up" and "basic to serve receive" so all can learn to move as a unit. Once players have a general sense of understanding of when this is used and how they adjust and set up, the coach may add the next step, getting from serve receive to offense, to hitter coverage, to defense. Players learn best when they are echoing or even saying the transition out loud as a team. The coach may add a toss and have players begin to "play it out." The coach may also introduce a lesson on overlapping, since players immediately in front and behind cannot overlap or have their feet cross each other, prior to the contact of the serve. Reminder: always return to basic before asking your players to rotate. Teach the lesson of being responsible for knowing which players are in front of you and behind you in rotation.

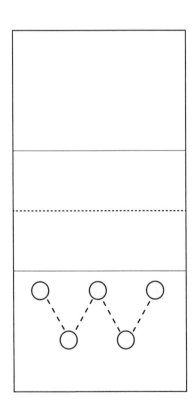 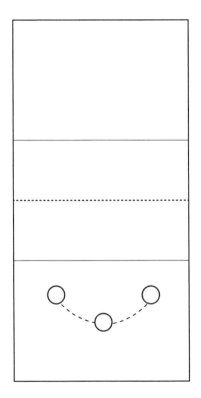

Cues

– No overlapping
– "Basic to adjust"

Serve Receive Formations:
– The "W": five players
– The Cup: three to four players

Number of Players: All

Player Positions: 6 vs 6 Formation

Instructions

The basic middle-back defense has only a few adjustments that players can learn to transition from hitter coverage to defense with a sense of confidence. Players start in basic defense, three players in the front row, three in the back row. This can be done from three lines on the baseline and wash the drill up a line and under the net to teach a little faster with less standing for players. The coach can use tape to show basic and a second piece of tape to show the adjusted spot for diggers to cover and for hitters to become blockers. Players are encouraged to not just get close or nearby their transition spot but to be precisely to the spot. As the coach slaps the ball and yells out the transition, all the players yell out, "Adjust, adjust." The coach may introduce specialized players or positions and when they can move to their "home." In the middle back defense, the middle back (MB) player is the "lateral mover." They cover line and move to the right 6-10 feet on their adjustment and typically stay a little deeper in the floor. The right back (RB) player, the setter if your offense has them coming out of the back row, typically rushes in and gets low to dig tips or dinks. The right back sets up behind the block. The blocker (B) who is not in front of the hit is called the "release blocker" and releases low and quickly to dig and should straddle the 10' line with their 10 toes facing swinging hitter. The final back row player, the left back (LB) digger, adjusts to cross-court coverage. Her cue words for ideal positioning are "bottom to the corner," referring to the alignment with the very deep corner of the floor. Not deep in the corner but realistically positioning to receive most hits and therefore, get the most digs.

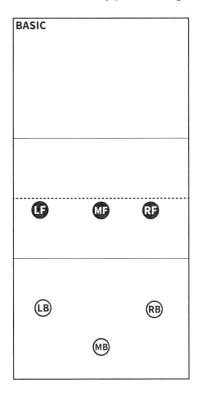

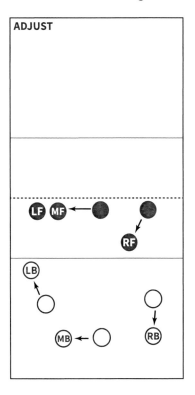

Cues

– Basic: "True to position"
– Adjust: "Adjust, adjust!"
– Always go back to basic before rotating players

Serve-A-Thon
Serving Drill

Number of Players: Two Groups

Player Positions: Baselines

Instructions

The coach divides the team into two even groups. These two serving teams start on the baseline with a volleyball, ready to serve. With five minutes on the clock, players realistically pledge out loud the number of serves they can successfully get in, both individually and as a team these projected numbers are set. The coach starts the drill and players quickly serve and go get another ball to serve doing their best to meet their realistic goal. The players may be under their projected number but cannot be over. If the player "pledged" 15 made serves in the five minute time allowed and they successfully make 16, then only the pledged number applies to their score. Players usually under pledge so they can feel certain to apply their score. Of course sportsmanship and honesty is quickly mentioned and the challenge is on! Players may figure out they can go get volleyballs for their teammates after they've reached their goal. See if they can figure out that strategy on their own! For a simpler, less competitive variation, have players pledge and get an entire team projected score and see what they ended up actually getting. Do the drill a second time being more realistic or raising the bar!

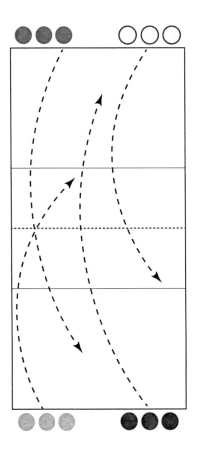

Cues

– Routine
– Teamwork
– Goal setting

Number of Players: Groups of Five to Seven

Player Positions: Circles

Instructions

Players are divided into two equal groups or the coach has all players in one large circle. All players communicate with the center circle player, who is the controlled pass or set between every circle touch. In other words, the axis starts the drill by tossing it to a teammate in the circle, they returns it back to the axis player and the team works to keep the ball up and alive, counting every touch as a point. Two teams can compete in a timed round or the team can simply try to beat their personal best score. Remind players to keep talking and stay low and active.

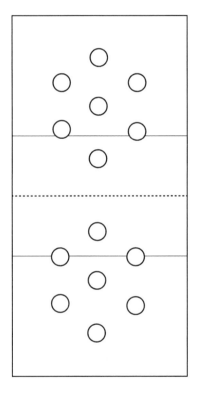

Cues

– Communicate
– Stay low
– Control is key!

REC+ Factor: Middle axis player is changed when coach yells, "New axis!" and two players have to quickly communicate, switch, and get in position for the next touch.

Belly Up and Switch
Passing Drill

Number of Players: All   **Player Positions:** Two Lines on Baseline

Instructions

Players are in two lines coming up from the baseline, facing the coach. This coach toss drill begins with the two players entering the floor belly down. Once the coach slaps the ball, both players pop up staying in a low ready-position and the coach tosses to one. The other immediately opens up and says, "go, go, go" as the passer "shovels" the ball back up to the coach/tosser. Immediately after that touch, the two players "switch, switch, switch" and the second passer gets that toss. They pass the ball back to the coach/tosser as the teammate opens and says, "go, go, go." Those two passers shag their volleyballs to the coach cart and return to the back of the line. Players should be talking the entire time and having active non-stop feet in the drill. Two good passes and two good communicators should "celebrate" as they dip under the net to shag. Enthusiasm makes this drill all the more exciting!

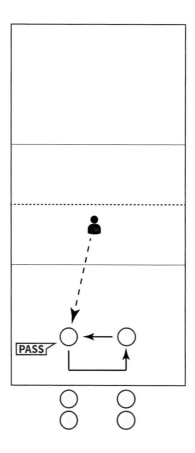

Cues

– "Pop to low"
– "Shovel" to target
– Communicate when switching
– One passes, both switch, second passes

Number of Players: Partners   **Player Positions:** 6 Stations Scattered

Instructions

The coach uses six station cards, file folders cut down and set up on edge or taped to cones, to identify six jump training exercises. The players are expected to work hard for the 30-45 seconds then jog between stations, clapping and demonstrating enthusiasm! The coach may demonstrate how hard work looks and what is expected for that short bout of time per each station.

The six stations are:

1) Front to back and side to side Jumps

2) Three step hitting approach

3) Lateral slides or lunges

4) Jump rope for speed

5) 1-2 blocking footwork: baby step, cross-over step, sit, and jump

6) 12' agility drill or some type of direction-changing challenge

Red, White, and Blue Hitting
Hitting Drill

Number of Players: All

Player Positions: Three Lines on Baseline

Instructions

This basic striking drill is about ball alignment on the hitting shoulder and learning to hit with an open hand. Players must ask for the ball by yelling, "Red, red, red!," "White, white, white!" or "Blue, blue, blue!" Once the coach hears them calling for the ball, the coach tosses a high toss. Players shuffle to get their shoulder lined up with the ball, point with their off-hand to the ball (track), and get into the trophy top pose. Stepping with the opposite foot and smacking the ball should be complete with a "firm finish," the statue pose at the end where the player is not falling off balance after contact.

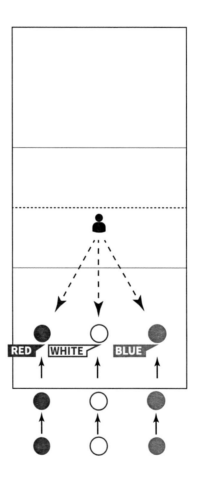

Cues

– Shoulder on ball
– High elbow
– Reach
– Trophy top
– Track and smack
– Finish firm

Number of Players: All

Player Positions: Hitting Lines

Instructions

Players are positioned in two lines angled to hit. Two jump ropes act as the alligator in the drill so that the alligator is directly in the 45° attack of the hitter. Players learn to **jump over the alligator** with a distinct step-close. The first step in our three step hitting approach is behind the alligator and jumping over the alligator is the step-close. Players then jump and the coach puts emphasis on **planting** the last part of the step close, listening for a squeak of the shoe. This plant step is to lock in the hitter's best **jumpers feet** so they may load and jump. Players head to the back of the line for another attempt. The coach can add a controlled toss once over the alligator for the players to get the feeling of jumping and contacting the ball. A full approach and swing with the alligator (ropes) may not be best, we wouldn't want hitters' feet getting tangled in the alligator!

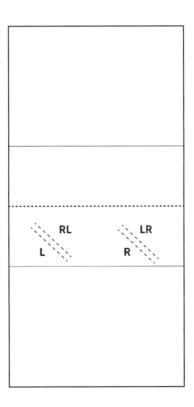

Cues

– Step, close over the alligator
– Strong plant foot to jump high
– Coach can add a toss

Pretzel
Passing Drill

Number of Players: Groups of Four   **Player Positions:** Group on Each Side of Net

Instructions

This drill has players in groups of four. There's a tosser with their back on the net and three passers about 15 feet out in front of the tosser. Like the look of a "Pretzel," players pass and switch with the player immediately next to them. The tosser switches up who they toss to. Passers stay **low** and open up to the other passers saying, "Go, go, go!" if it's not their ball. The player passing should always **claim** the ball, calling, "My ball, my ball, my ball!" If the ball is tossed to the middle passer, outside players must hold for a split-second as the middle passer picks who they will switch with. The pretzel-like movement continues until the coach yells out, "New tosser." This control passing drill can be timed for 30-45 seconds as the coach insists on staying low that entire time period.

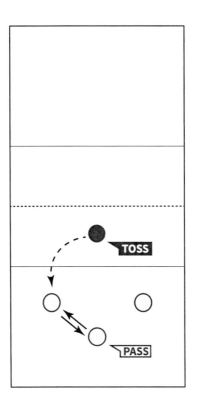

Cues

– Stay low
– Talk the entire time
– Celebrate at the end of each round
– After pass, passer switches with closest passer

Step and Stick
Defensive Drill

Number of Players: All

Player Positions: Two Lines on Baseline

Instructions

The cue phrase "step and stick" refers to the step toward the ball to get hips near the ball and the stick is sticking the platform out under the ball. This defense drill has players in two lines facing the coach. The two players step out to the floor, low and ready to step and stick. The ball contact should be low as the coach can control the intensity of the throw or down ball. The players dig their ball, shag it, and return it to the ball cart before heading back to their digging lines. The coach may say, "All digs will be to your right" or "All digs will be to your left" to give players a sense of quick success with less reading or having to guess where the ball with fall.

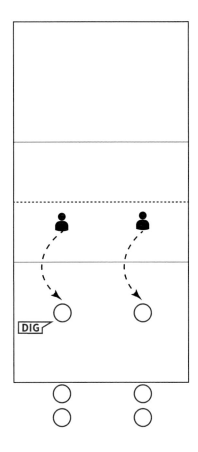

Cues

– "Step and stick"
– "Lengthen to the ball"
– "Hands to the floor"
– "Drop net shoulder"

Serve and Sprint
Serving Drill

Number of Players: Individual

Player Positions: Baseline

Instructions

Divide the team in half with each half on the serving baselines. Learning to "gain composure" after exertion, players serve and sprint to the opposite serving line. They reset their feet, take a deep breath, and start their routine. Once the player serves they practice calming down and being an effective server. The coach may put a certain amount of time on this challenge.

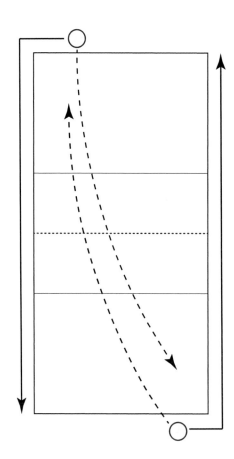

Cues

– Server's composure
– Exaggerate a deep breath to relax before serving

REC+ Factor: Conditioning drill, followed by composure

Free Ball, Free Ball, Free Ball, Attack
Team Drill

Number of Players: All

Player Positions: Three Lines on Baseline

Instructions

Two coaches are ideal so that there are volleyballs coming from both outside hitting areas. The players are placed in a 6 vs 6 formation, three lines on the baseline is ideal if the team is large enough. The 6 vs 6 set up allows for a scrimmage-like feel and players rehearse transitioning from defense to offense on a free ball. Once the ball is dead, the other coach sends a free ball to the other side and after a third free ball, the final transition is a hard-driven down ball. The team tries to turn this dig into an offense, hitter coverage, then finally back to defense. Players communicate each transition loudly by yelling, "defense-defense, cover-cover, free-free." The coach can wash the drill or have players rotate a position to ensure all players are familiar with all positions and duties.

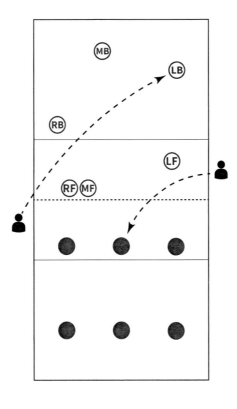

Cues

– 6 vs 6
– Always moving
– Always talking

REC+ Factor: An attack from one coach can be changed into an "adjusted" defense, play all balls out

Volleyball Jog
Warm-up Drill

Number of Players: All

Player Positions: Around Court

Instructions

The players go for a light and easy jog around the floor - as a team! With a ball under their arm, players stop on coaches whistle and as they "rest" they perform a series of ball handling challenges such as popcorn, down balls, and self-sets. Once a challenge is over, players go another lap or two awaiting the whistle for their next task. This is a good ball handling activity.

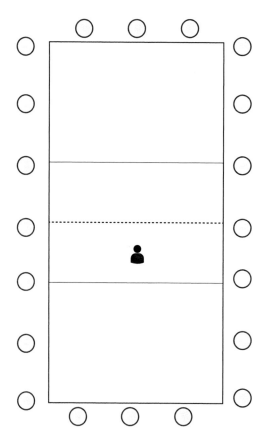

Cues

– Team jogs around the court
– Big and soft hands when setting
– Long and strong arms when passing

Coach stops team to perform challenges:

– Popcorn
– Self-sets
– Low passing catches
– Floor down balls

Number of Players: Individual

Player Positions: On Wall

Instructions

All players have a ball and are positioned on a wall approximately 10-15 feet away. All players are back in **Year One**! Each time a player successfully has a wall down ball: hand, floor, wall, hand, floor, wall, they move up to the next year. The goal is to graduate with 12 consecutive contacts and then off to college, grad school, PhD, and off to the **Olympics**! The Olympics may result in a Gold, Silver, or Bronze medal depending on the criteria set by the coach. For example: Bronze medal could be 30 in-a-row, Silver 35, Gold 50 or more!

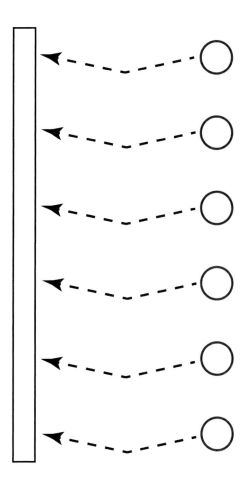

Cues

– Players start at Year One
– For each consecutive down ball, players gain a year
– If a player misses, they go back to Year One to start

8 in 8
Serving Drill

Number of Players: All

Player Positions: Serving Baselines

Instructions

Players are divided equally on both service baselines. In eight attempts, counted out by the coach, players work hard to successfully serve eight **consecutive** volleyballs over the net and in! This may not happen the first time! It's a good team goal. Players should be reminded how to act and treat one another when teammates miss a serve. This can be modeled for them and emphasized as a way of dealing with player mess ups! **All players** are working together as the coach counts the good serves. Eight serves in eight minutes may work better for some initial success if eight attempts is too tough.

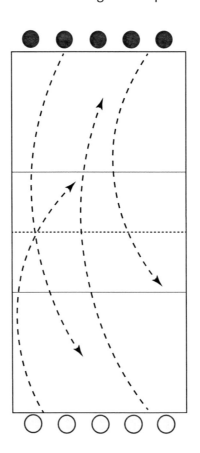

Cues

– Stay calm
– Deep breath before each serve
– Do your routine each time

Number of Players: Individual

Player Positions: Serving Baselines

Instructions

With players equally serving along both baselines the coach calls out the exertion exercise and immediately following that exercise, players serve. Players should be reminded to start their routine, remembering to breathe and get in a confident state of mind! The coach can allow a certain amount of time for the drill or set the goal of a certain number of made serves.

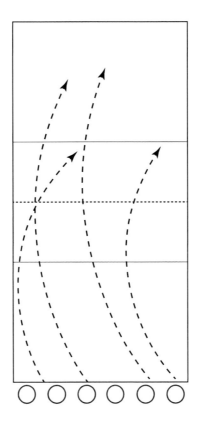

Exertion Exercise

– Push-ups
– Sit-ups
– Burpees
– Running
– Explosion jumps

REC+ Factor: Players are asked to visualize the score being 24-23 with us in the lead and we need a serve to finish! Or players can visualize we have 23 points and we need two serves to finish!

Dig One, Serve One
Defensive, Serving Drill

Number of Players: All

Player Positions: One Line on Baseline

Instructions

With players in a digging line and the coach on the net to toss, players begin with a dig and quickly step out to serve. Two players are across the net to serve receive. While one passer claims the ball, "My ball, my ball!" the other passer opens up and says, "Go, go, go!" Players rotate from being a back row **digger to server to a passer** or the coach can have players stay in that assigned position until the coach calls out rotate. Cue words such as "step and stick" are used to dig, while the serving routine cues are used, along with the passers saying, "1, 2, freeze" to get in "hips to the ball" receiving position.

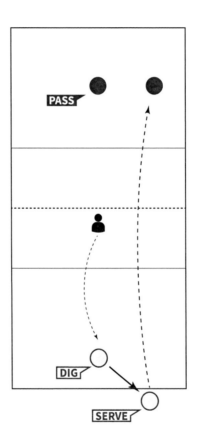

Cues

- Players dig and then hustle out immediately to serve
- **Dig:** "Step and stick"
- **Serve:** "Composure"
- **Pass**: "1, 2, freeze"

Number of Players: All

Player Positions: Net to Baseline

Instructions

Players set up like they are beginning a partner drill with one partner with their back on the net, the other on the baseline. The players at the net are the tossers and the players near the baseline are the setters. Tossers slap the ball and give an "It's up!" call on the coach's whistle. All players do this at the same time. High tosses to the setters will allow them to **draw** their hands, establish strong "setter's feet" and extend, holding their follow-through. Setters then all rotate, never walking, to the next tosser. Remember to switch up your tossers and setters so all players get their setting touches. Going off the coach's whistle will keep the drill organized and allow for a sense of excellence!

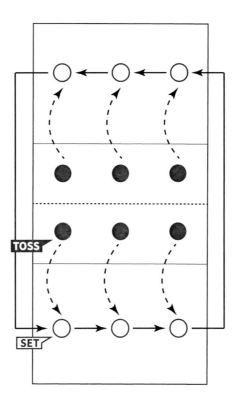

Cues

– Feet first
– Draw hands
– Shuffle on the run
– Strong follow through and hold

REC+ Factor: Speed up the drill and make the players move faster.

Set the Setter
Passing, Setting, Hitting Drill

Number of Players: All

Player Positions: Passer, Setter, and Two Hitters

Instructions

In this drill the coach tosses over the net to a passer, the passer will **set** to the setter and the hitter will swing away! The setter may have **two hitters** in place: a middle attacker and an outside. The setter can practice **calling their set** by saying which hitter they are setting. Players will rotate after every touch or many times it's better to rotate after a series of attempts.

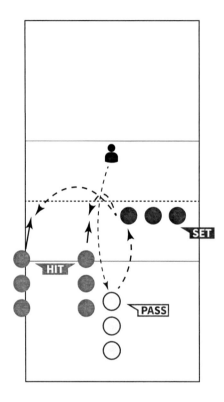

Cues

– Passers work on taking the ball overhand
– Start hitters on the net
– **Transition footwork:** "Drop, cross, hop, hop"

Number of Players: All

Player Positions: 6 Players on the Court

Instructions

Players are positioned on one side of the net in a defensive digging formation, middle back defense perhaps. Players adjust on the coach's ball slap from **basic to defense** and get a dig. 10 to Win simply means that 10 digs or ups, for beginners, will result in coming out of the drill or a rotation of players to a new position. Blockers can still learn to jump and "release" off the net as they land. A "touch-help" is emphasized when the blockers have contact with the ball. Remind diggers to stay low as they adjust and not to move tall and then drop to low!

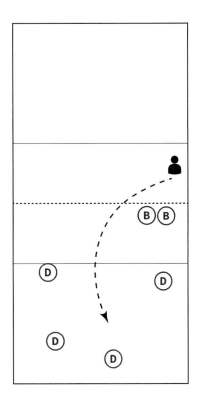

Cues

– 10 digs from four digging positions working for 10 playable ups
– **Blockers**: "Touch" or "Help"
– May introduce the Libero position
– **Diggers**: "Step and stick"

Won It, Lost It, Tied It
Serving Drill

Number of Players: All

Player Positions: Baselines

Instructions

The score is 23-24 and we are down. Players, half on each baseline, are asked to serve **two** balls. Players complete their serving routine and serve one and then the next. Depending on the two serves and whether they made them or not depends on whether the individual player "Won it," "Lost it," or "Tied it." Meaning, players serve two total serves and if they made only one they "Tied it" but if they miss both serves they "Lost it." A player can of course "Win it" by serving two back to back serves successfully over the net. Players just yell out the outcome of their serves and go right into the next two serves. This is a good opportunity for the coach to remind players they must be able to maintain or regain composure after a let down, when they "Lost it." It also teaches a lesson on accountability!

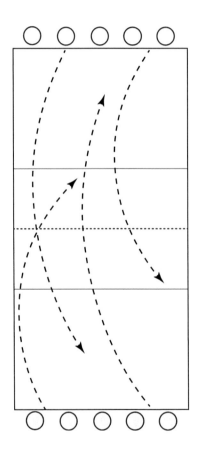

Cues

- Score is 23-24 and we are down
- Players have two serves to win the game
- **"Won It"**- made both serves
- **"Tied It"**- made one, missed one
- **"Lost It"**- missed both serves
- Routine and rhythm

Number of Players: Partners

Player Positions: Net to Baseline

Instructions

Players are partnered up factoring in skill level. Partners pepper using the cue words: **toss, pass, set, down ball, dig**. When players perform all five skills in-a-row, from the toss to the dig, the players yell out the **pepper** they accomplished or earned. For example, partners just peppered so the first time they accomplish this they yell out "Bell pepper," the second successful round they yell out, "Banana pepper," etc. Once a couple pairs get to the ghost pepper, the coach can throw out a **Carolina Reaper Pepper** challenge, three in-a-row non-stop peppers. Players are reminded to extend on their set then recover low to dig and to always **recover** back to the general area after each touch.

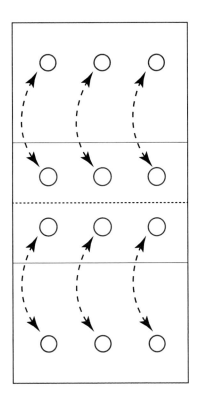

Cues

Peppers:
- One Pepper: Bell
- Two peppers: Banana
- Three peppers: Jalapeño
- Four peppers: Habanero
- Five peppers: Ghost

Line Shuttle Drill
Passing, Setting Drill

Number of Players: Groups of Five or Six   **Player Positions:** Two Lines Facing the Other

Instructions

The coach divides the team into two even line facing one another with the first player in each line ready to pass or set. Starting with a toss across to the player in line, the first person passes or sets back to the line the ball started. After contact, players immediately run to the line they passed or set to. In other words, players pass or set and run to the back of the other line. This Shuttle Line keeps track of the number of consecutive touches. Coaches can challenge the team or lines to a personal team best or have two lines compete against one another. Also, adding time to the drill can challenge players to the number of no mess ups. A high pass or set allows for players to get in position for more success.

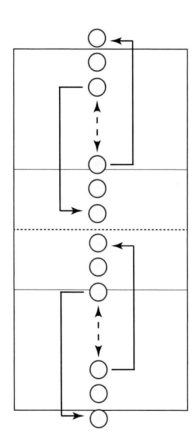 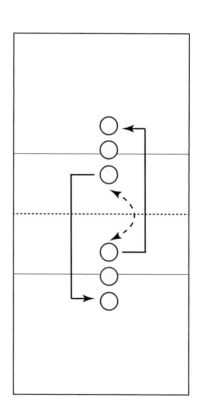

Cues

– Tosser chases their own toss to begin
– Passers follow their pass and join the back of the other line
– Feet first, then freeze
– "High buy times"
– Communication is key!

Number of Players: All

Player Positions: Baselines

Instructions

The coach divides the group in two and places one group on each of the two baselines. Players work hard to serve three short serves (2-3-4 serving zones) followed by three deep serves (1, 6, 5 serving zones). The coach can vary the serving zone calls, for example two deep, one short.

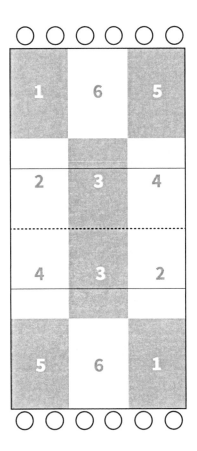

Cues

- Short serves: 2, 3, 4
- Long serves: 1, 6, 5
- Coach can vary the number of short and deep serves
- Routine and rhythm

Hit and Exit
Hitting Drill

Number of Players: All   **Player Positions:** Six Hitters on Net

Instructions

The coach sets up three or four chairs along both sides of the net. In unison, players release off the net with their solid footwork, drop, cross, hop, hop, and swing at the same time. The catch is that they must exit, slide over and behind the chair, and then move as a unit to swing. As one player shuffles out the end of the drill past the last chair, they run behind the drill to get back in line. The drill looks great when it's done in unison, somewhat dance-like. Players are encouraged to call out the **designated** numbers or calls. Correct footwork, arm swings, and communication are key in making this a smooth and fun drill.

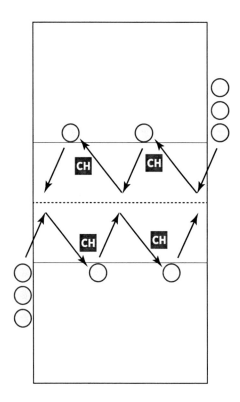

Cues

– Transition footwork: "Drop, cross, hop, hop"

Hitting Calls:
– Outside: "4, 4, 4!"
– Middle: "2, 2, 2!"
– Right Side: "C, C, C!"

Number of Players: All

Player Positions: 6 vs 6

Instructions

Players are set up 6 vs 6. From a coach's toss, over the net, players receive a free ball and play it out to **cover**, hitter coverage, as they call out, "Cover, cover, cover!" The players across from them stay active and call out "Down, down, down!" as they prepare to dig the returned ball. The coach may rotate players or wash the drill depending on numbers. A strong "It's up!" call reminds teammates that the ball is live and we are in offense with the goal of three hits!

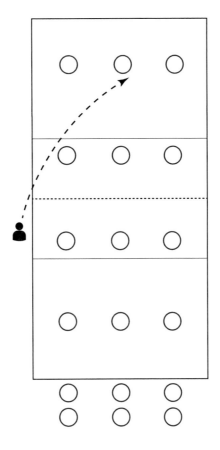

Cues

Team yells:
- "Down, down, down!"
- "Cover, cover, cover!"
- "It's up!"
- "Defense, defense!"

Jail Break
Serving Drill

Number of Players: All

Player Positions: Service Line

Instructions

All players serve from the Law Abiding Citizens side of the net. When a serve is missed the player who missed is "off to jail." There are two ways a player can get out of jail: coach yells "Jail break!" or a player claims a serve and catches it. If a player catches the volleyball from jail, they go back to the serving side and the player whose ball was caught goes to jail! This classic drill is always a team favorite.

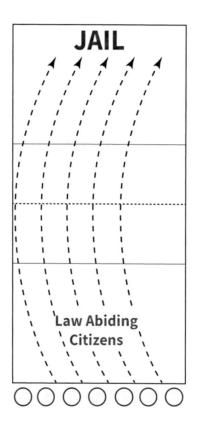

Cues

– Routine to punch
– **Good serve:** keep serving
– **Miss:** off to jail
– **Ticket out of jail:** catch a served ball
– **Serve is caught:** off to jail
– Coach may call "Jail break!" to free all

Number of Players: All   **Player Positions:** Scattered on Half the Floor

Instructions

All volleyball players report to the spiderweb! The web is on one side of the floor anywhere inbounds but behind the 10' line. Coach picks a couple of "serving spiders" to begin serving the spider eggs (volleyballs) over the net into the web full of spiders. When a serving spider hits a spider directly, that spider becomes a serving spider. Make sure players are facing the serving spiders and they cover their heads if a spider egg looks like it's going to hit them above the shoulders. When all spiders are serving and the game is down to the last two or three spiders, the non-serving spiders become the new serving spiders, starting a new game. Spiders cannot move unless the coach yells out "Spider shuffle!" then the spiders all jump up, dance the spider dance, and return to the web after the serving spiders go shag all the volleyballs - of course, we mean spider eggs!

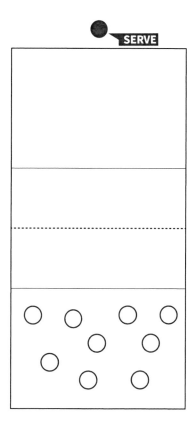

Cues

– Goal: have all spiders serving to get that last spider
– A direct hit "frees" the hit spider to serve
– Do not allow the spiders to be in front of the 10 ft line

Free Ball, Free Ball, Free Ball, Wash
Team Drill

Number of Players: All   **Player Positions:** Three Lines on Baseline

Instructions

Players line up in three lines on the baseline. Players are sent out to the court in a "wash" drill formation, playing 6 vs 6, or 3 vs 3 if there are not enough players. The coach tosses over the net to the side **opposite** from the three lines. From the toss the players play volleyball. After three free ball tosses from the coach, players all yell "Wash!" and players rotate up the floor. When players wash off the court they shag their three volleyballsand return to their lines. An uneven number works fine, the players file in as they come back around the floor to the 3LoBL. The team goal and goal for every player should be to be "always talking and always moving."

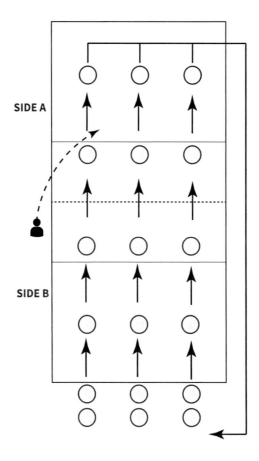

Cues

– three free ball tosses form the coach
– After three free balls have been played out, wash
– 6 vs 6 or 3 vs 3
– Always talking
– Always moving

Number of Players: Partners   **Player Positions:** Partners at a Station

Instructions

These eight jump training stations are quite the workout! Have partners work hard at these eight stations.

The eight stations are:

1) Plyo step-close

2) 12' agility drill (pg.112)

3) Jump rope

4) 1-2 middle blocker footwork

5) One-step candy cane jumps (blocker candy canes hands up and over the net - straight up and back down)

6) Agility ladder work

7) One leg bounding (long skipping - skipping for height not length)

8) Two foot explosive ups.

Players should stay in the station for 30 seconds minimum and focus on good technique and speed reps. Players are expected to be enthusiastic and support one another between stations. Remind players to rotate with a jog and to never walk!

Down Ball Net Work
Ball Control Drill

Number of Players: Partners   **Player Positions:** Partners Across Net

Instructions

Players will have a partner and be across the net from one another, a giant step behind the 10' line. Players will go on the coach's call for the various **net** challenges:

1) Net Down Balls: Ball only gets to bounce once and go over or under the net
2) Net Tiny Passes: The partners will pass **under** the net, needing to keep the ball low and platforms ready
3) Net Digs: Partners will down ball to one another and dig as the ball travels under the net
4) Net Sets: This touch is above the net, setting back and forth over for consecutive partner touches

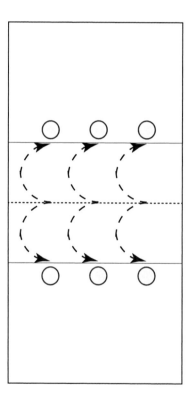

Cues

– Controlled touches
– Communicate contacts

REC+ Factor: Coach hits the whistle quick, 30-45 seconds, switching skills fast and emphasizing to the players to **not** visit between challenges but instead figure things out with body language and precise volleyball communication.

Number of Players: Groups of Three or Four   **Player Positions:** Each Group at a Station

Instructions

These four stations are perfect for muscle-memory repetition:

1) Noodle Reaches: Using half a pool noodle, players reach with a high elbow and step with the opposite foot to hit the basketball net

2) Hoop Toss: Players toss the volleyball to the bottom of the basketball net

3) Wall Pins and Tosses: Players toss or deliver the ball to the ideal height and **pin** it to the wall, the ball should travel straight up and down the wall and not **jumbo shrimp** back!

4) Mock Serving Drill: Players grabs a partner and control serve from 10' line to 10' line over the net

 Coaches - ideally, players can train at these stations for four to five minutes each. Players will rotate on the coaches call or whistle.

Mock Serving
Serving Drill

Number of Players: Partners   **Player Positions:** Partners Across Net

Instructions

Partners are across the net from one another starting at the 10' line. The receiving partner is a big target with hands up, ready to catch. Serving partner is focused on the details of serving as coach places emphasis and reminders on the toss, the ball alignment, the punch, etc. Players are asked to take one step back after a few minutes of serving.

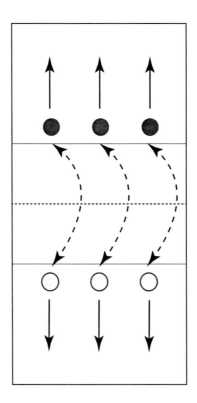

Cues

Overhand:
– Toss, step, punch
– Elbow by the eye
– Finish firm

Underhand:
– Ball on shoulder
– Drip of sweat
– 1, 2, punch

Number of Players: All

Player Positions: Three Lines on Baseline

Instructions

Players are positioned in three lines on the baseline. The coach is on the same side of the players with the cart and volleyballs. With six players on the floor, the coach slaps the ball and says "It's up!" The coach's toss is the first hit, meaning the side of six only has 2 more contacts to get the ball over the net. The coach's toss is a "bad pass" and the next two hits are the "good save." This drill is a real game-like drill. It helps prepare the team for a less-than-great first pass. The second hit or first save should be brought back to the middle of the floor so the team can call out the third hit. The team must survive the bad pass and make something good come out of things. The three diggers on the other side of the net help shag and may play it out, if time permits. Players rotate on the wash call by the coach. Passers move up to the front row, the front row dips under the net and become the new diggers, the old diggers shag any balls that are out then hop back in line.

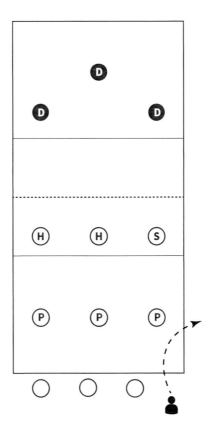

Cues

– 6 vs 3 wash dril
– Coach's toss is the first contact
– The team of six has two more contacts to get the ball over the net
– Run and hustle to ball with "runner's arms"

Back Row Attacks to Defense
Hitting Drill

Number of Players: All

Player Positions: 4 vs 4

Instructions

Coaches will set players up 4 vs 4. A coach will toss the ball from the back row to the setter and the setter will set a **red, white, or blue**. The setter can call the back row set or the coach can call the shots. Players are encouraged to **ask** for the ball by yelling the appropriate call and the back row hitter can hit or down ball over the net. The coach may determine if the ball is to be played out or the drill alternates from side to side. Players want to "cover" the hit by dropping down in a digging posture and say "Cover, cover!" as the hitter swings and attacks. Rotate the drill by sliding players over a position and eventually all will have a turn to be the setter.

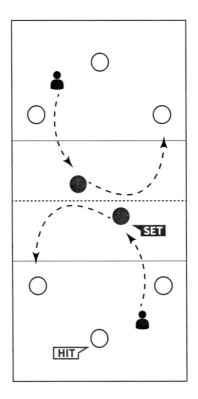

Cues

– Coach tosses to setter from the same side
– Back row attacks only
– Back row hitters should ask for their set: "Red," "White," or "Blue"

Number of Players: All

Player Positions: Three Lines on Baseline

Instructions

Players line up in three lines on the baseline while coach is across the net from the Queen side with a cart of volleyballs. First player in each line are the Queens (Q). As the Queens dip under the net to find the Royal Courtyard, the Princesses (P) step on to challenge them. The coach always tosses across the net to the Queen side. If either side attempts three hits by passing a controlled pass up to the setter's zone, the coach grants a life and that team gets a "do over." A life is a way to emphasize three hits volleyball. When a play ends, new Challengers (CH) come onto the floor and either the Queens remain (Queens won the point) or new Queens run under the net to take over (Princesses won the point). Whichever side lost the point always shags the volleyball and returns to their lines. For an uneven number of players encourage new partners.

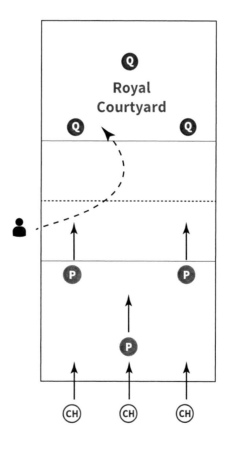

Cues

– Queens receive ball
– Call, "Free ball!" on coach's slap
– **Earn a life:** pass goes to setter zone
– **Queens win point:** Queens stay, Challengers step on
– **Princesses win point:** Queens off, Princesses move to Queen side, Challengers step on

Speed Hitting
Hitting Drill

Number of Players: All

Instructions

Less talking and coaching and more swinging! Players are organized in three hitting lines: Outside, Middle, Right Side. Players **hit, shag, and return** to the lines. Coaches remind players to line up, quickly get to the ball, draw their arms early, and be in **attack mode**! The coach may add a clock to the drill and have someone count successful hits. Hit and hustle is the theme! Players should return to the shortest line and not always hit from their favorite position. Lots of enthusiasm and celebrating of big hits will help the drill be effective and fun!

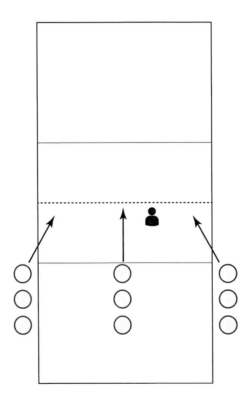

Cues

– Coach tosses
– Hitters hit, shag, and return to line
– Time the drill and count number of hits
– Hit and hustle

Number of Players: All

Player Positions: Line of Setters

Instructions

Setters line up in right back ready to hustle to the setting zone. Once the setter gets to the net they move left. Either six "targets" or players can be in the designated areas. The coach can call out, prior to the toss, the target or setters can attempt to set to all six spots! Players rotate on as the setter rotates off to shag or return to the line. The coach emphasizes the right foot slightly forward and the weight transfer out to that front leg as the setter lengthens and extends.

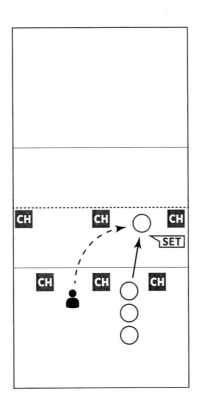

Cues

– Setter footwork: "Left jab, right plant" and "Plant and pivot"
– Get to the net and then move left
– Setters targets can be players who can free ball the ball over
– Setters targets can be objects, for example: trash cans, hula hoops, chairs, or cones

Tennis Ball Touch
Defensive Drill

Number of Players: All

Player Positions: Three Lines on Baseline or Partners

Instructions

From either three lines on the baseline or with partners, players toss a tennis ball expecting the digger to **reach and touch** the ball. Players "step and stick" toward the tennis ball, say "I go!" and work hard to get the touch. The coach can count touches or simply let players work to meet the touch challenge. Players will switch or rotate every 1-2 minutes per coach's whistle. An emphasis will be to encourage diggers to drop low and watch the ball fall nearly to the floor before committing to touch it. The coach should review safety measures such as how to go to the floor safely and how to reach and lengthen to the ball.

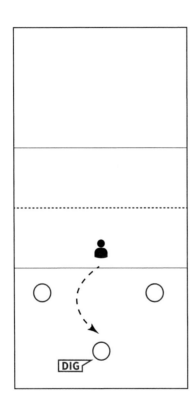 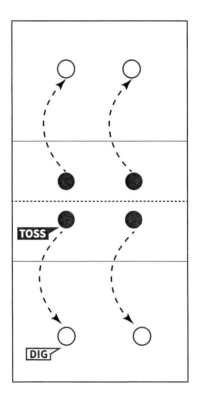

Cues

– Step and stick
– "I go!"
– "Touch, touch!"
– Players drop to low hips and dig or touch every ball

Number of Players: All

Player Positions: Three Hitters vs Four Diggers

Instructions

Three hitters vs. four diggers formation will allow the defense to adjust so that they are able to cover and dig. The coach can place four defenders in basic and adjust to the three hitters attacking angles. The coach will toss to the hitters and the diggers will play it out. Players can rotate through on defense and the hitters can also switch hitting positions.

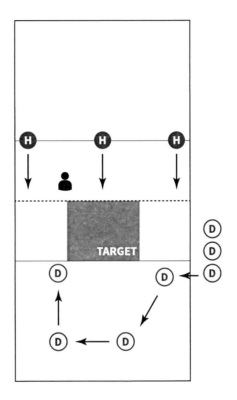

Cues

– Focus on large setter's zone
– "Step and stick"
– Low platforms and low hands
– "It's up!"

REC+ FACTOR: Rotate diggers after three digs, a great dig = 3 Points, a good dig = 2 Points, and an over pass results in a -1 from the digger's total. The coach can define the setter's zone using a King-size sheet, cones, taped area, or a gym mat.

Speed Ball
Team Drill

Number of Players: Groups of Three or Four   **Player Positions:** Three or Four Lines on Baseline

Instructions

Lines on the baseline will organize players for either 3 vs 3 play or 4 vs 4 play. Every touch is a point. The coach puts the ball in play with a free ball and players earn up to 3 points on one side, but the ball could be returned for additional points. Players play the free ball toss until it's defined dead and the players wash. The free ball toss always goes to side A. Players keep the **same teammates**.

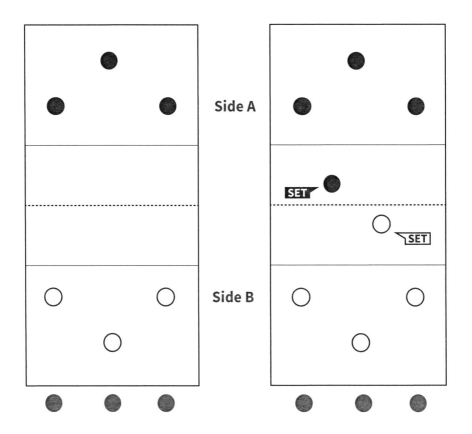

Cues

– 4 vs 4 wash
– Every touch is a point
– A touch is any contact with effort

REC+ Factor: a true three hits play where the hit goes over the net can result in a bonus 2 points, so the team would get 5 points instead of 3. The winning team does three push-ups while the non-winning team does 5 push-ups. The coach can reshuffle players and play another round!

Year Six

Year Six players are in full three hit volleyball mode! Players work in groups of three, and in tons of partner drills. The name of the game, to insist on perfecting fundamental skill sets, is exaggerate.

Players will hold their follow-through to "look like high school athletes" when they demonstrate skills, and transition on and off the net with a general understanding of an offense. Players will be "invested in the details" with quick cue-words and phrase driven language. Players will be expected to show great form and mechanics with the overhand serve and demonstrate the full three step or four step hitting approach. The emphasis should be placed on the form and technique and not the end result.

Add lots of wash drills to mix the team up and be mindful of keeping all encouraged as this is a big time when volleyball loses kids. Identifying a setter and how to serve-receive and making floor position adjustments with your players will be a big lesson for your team. Players have many years up ahead of specialization, so working to have players in all positions may be the most positive approach.

Year 6

Practice Schedule
Year Six

	Page	**Drill**
Week 4	193	Early Bird Special
	206	Jump Train x6
	212	Serve and Sprint
	213	Shuffle Back Passing
	247	Lesson: Sprawling
	214	Touch Two
	215	Shuffle, Shuffle, Freeze "Dance"
	216	Butterfly
	217	Attacks vs Digs
Week 5	193	Early Bird Special
	218	Wall Work Series
	194	Dynamic Warm-up
	195	Team Stretch
	196	Four Muscle Memory Throws
	219	Speedball
	213	Shuffle Back Pass
	251	Serving the Setter and Sub
	220	Jump Training x6
	221	Agility and Vertical Jump
Week 6	193	Early Bird Special
	250	Jump Rope
	194	Dynamic Warm-up
	195	Team Stretch
	196	Four Muscle Memory Throws
	222	Four Corners
	209	Spot Serving
	223	Transition Volleyball Drill
	224	3 Deep
	251	Serve Receive to Finish
	241	Personal Best Score Card (Year 4-6)

Practice Schedule
Year Six

Number of Players: All   **Player Positions:** Scattered

Instructions

The Early Bird Special (EBS) is all about hitting the ground running. Players get a ball immediately upon entering the gym and begin their EBS routine or the warm-up. Players stay engaged and repeat until the coach brings the full group together. The EBS should end the question, "what do we do?" as players arrive.

Example 1

1. Jog two laps
2. 20 floor down balls
3. 20 wall sets
4. 20 self-bumps
5. 10 wall serves

Example 2

1. 25 jumping Jills
2. 5 push ups
3. 20 wall serves
4. Pepper with a pal

Example 3

1. 50 popcorns
2. 50 self-sets
3. 50 down balls

Example 4

1. 20 net jumps
2. 30 partner passes and sets
3. 40 line runs

Cues

– Same or different challenges
– Serves as you warm-up
– Reviews and reinforces skills
– Immediate touches

Year 6

Dynamic Warm-up
Warm-up Drill

Number of Players: All

Player Positions: Three Lines on Baseline

Instructions

Dynamic warm-up includes a series of stretches from high knees to bottom kicks. Players line up in three lines on the baseline and on the coach's whistle are brought out from their lines. Players can do the warm-up exercise to the net and back, with lots of high-fives and enthusiasm as they return to the line. Coach can emphasize players being **attentive** and **invested** in the details and remind the players to "lift toes," "drive the knee," "keep shoulders parallel with the wall," etc.

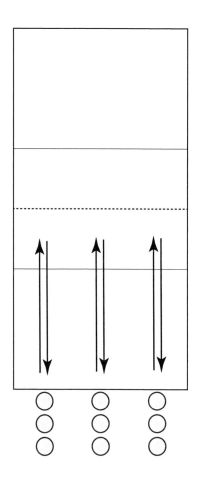

Suggested Exercises

- High knee with a skip
- Bounds with a skip
- Butt kickers
- Grapevine
- Frankensteins
- Jogging, forwards and backwards

Number of Players: All

Player Positions: Lines

Instructions

The team is in lines, orderly and uniform. As the coach moves players through a series of static stretches the players stay involved and engaged by counting and holding the stretches. The coach yells out the **odd** numbers as the players count the **even** numbers. Players either clap two times or slap the floor two times after the 10 count and chant their team name!

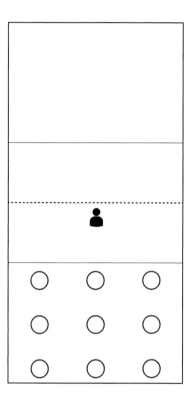

Suggested Stretches

– RT over LT
– LT over RT
– Straddle
– Arm front and behind stretches
– Butterfly and hurdle stretch

Four Muscle Memory Throws
Warm-up Drill

___

Number of Players: Partners

Player Positions: Net to Baseline

Instructions

There are four muscle-memory throws:

1) Two Thumbs by the Thighs - players, positioned with a partner, throw for warm-up and also for developing essential movements in overhand serving, hitting, and hip rotation. Two Thumbs by the Thighs has partners bouncing the ball hard once to the floor - playing catch - back and forth.

2) Elbow by the Eye - players pause and adjust their throwing arm to get the throwing arm elbow "by the eye." As they throw with the opposite foot forward, the coach reminds players of the opening and closing of their hips. Players throw from high to low, meaning wrist snap at the release, aiming for the receiving partners knee pads.

3) Back to Your Partner - partners face away from their partner and step forward, with either foot to switch it up, arching the back and "throwing their chest to the ceiling" and holding their arms way up high pose.

4) Two Slaps and a Down Ball - two big open hand "slappy" sounds on the ball followed by a down ball to their partner. The ball bounces once. Remind players in this "throw" to not toss the ball but hit it out of their own hand or after a very small toss.

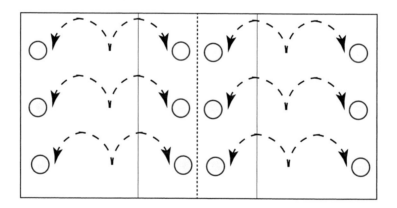

Cues

Throws:

1) Two Thumbs by the Thigh	Hard throws to the floor
2) Elbow by the Eye	Elbow starts high and leads
3) Back to Your Partner	Big and animated
4) Two Slaps and a Down Ball	Slaps with elbow lead

Dig 'Em Up
Defensive Drill

Number of Players: All

Player Positions: Two Lines on Baseline

Instructions

Players are in two even lines. The coach has their back on the net and alternates tosses between the two lines of diggers. **Every time** a dig gets up the team earns 3 points. If a ball hits the floor the team loses a point. The team works hard to "step and stick" and contact the ball with "low hands." The coach sets the goal, for example, 18 points for the drill to end.

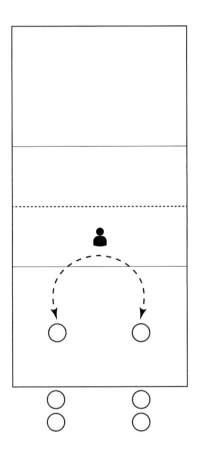

Cues

– Dig: +3
– Ball hits floor: -1
– "Step and stick"
– "Low hands"

REC+ Factor: Players are expected to get to their knee pads, lengthen to the ball for the touch and find the floor when needed! Players dig, shag, and return to the drill lines.

Pepper
Passing, Setting, Hitting Drill

Number of Players: Partners

Player Positions: Net to Baseline

Instructions

Players are partnered up factoring in skill level. Partners pepper using the cue words: **toss, pass, set, down ball, dig**. When players perform all five skills in-a-row, from the toss to the dig, the players yell out the **pepper** they accomplished or earned. For example, partners just peppered so the first time they accomplish this they yell out "Bell pepper," the second successful round they yell out, "Banana pepper," etc. Once a couple pairs get to the ghost pepper, the coach can throw out a **Carolina Reaper Pepper** challenge, three in-a-row non-stop peppers. Players are reminded to extend on their set then recover low to dig and to always **recover** back to the general area after each touch.

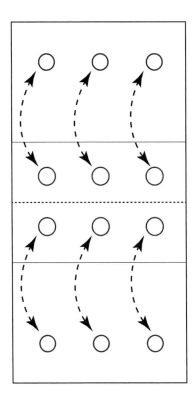

Peppers

– One pepper: Bell
– Two peppers: Banana
– Three peppers: Jalapeño
– Four peppers: Habanero
– Five peppers: Ghost

Number of Players: Groups of Three

Player Positions: 2 Passers Near Baseline and Tosser at the Net

Instructions

The coach arranges players in groups of three with one tosser and two passers. The tosser has their back on the net. The tosser tosses the same course with each and every toss. The two passers are side by side. The first passer passes back to the tosser and both passers **quickly**, "Switch, switch, switch!" The passer who passes the ball back to the tosser claims the volleyball by saying, "My ball, my ball!" and the non-passer, **opens up** and says, "Go, go, go!" The coach calls out new tosser to rotate players. Keeping players in the drill for 30-45 seconds will place emphasis on being a low and ready passer. In this drill, **all players** are talking and communicating.

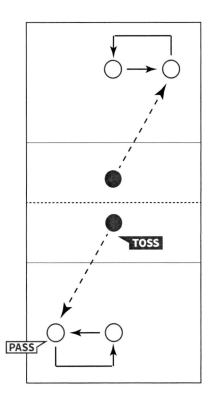

Cues

– Tosser tosses to the same spot every toss
– Passers switch with each pass
– **Players need to talk:**
– "Switch, switch, switch!"
– "My ball!"
– "Go, go, go!"

Queens of the Court
Team Drill

Number of Players: All   **Player Positions:** Three Lines on Baseline

Instructions

Players line up in three lines on the baseline while coach is across the net from the Queen side with a cart of volleyballs. First player in each line are the Queens (Q). As the Queens dip under the net to find the Royal Courtyard, the Princesses (P) step on to challenge them. The coach always tosses across the net to the Queen side. If either side attempts three hits by passing a controlled pass up to the setter's zone, the coach grants a life and that team gets a "do over." A life is a way to emphasize three hits volleyball. When a play ends, new Challengers (CH) come onto the floor and either the Queens remain (Queens won the point) or new Queens run under the net to take over (Princesses won the point). Whichever side lost the point always shags the volleyball and returns to their lines. For an uneven number of players encourage new partners.

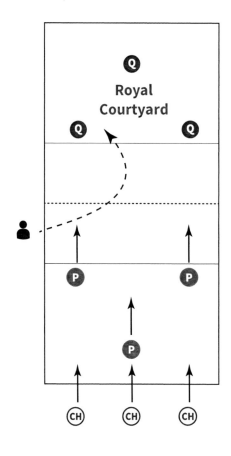

Cues

– Queens receive ball
– Call, "Free ball!" on coach's slap
– **Earn a life:** pass goes to setter zone
– **Queens win point:** Queens stay, Challengers step on
– **Princesses win point:** Queens off, Princesses move to Queen side, Challengers step on

Toss, Pass, Perfection Ups
Passing Drill

Number of Players: Partners

Player Positions: Net to Baseline

Instructions

Players have a partner and are positioned on the floor with one back on the net and the other on the baseline. The player with their back on the net is the tosser and slaps the ball and calls out "It's up!" The passer passes the ball back to the tosser. The tosser can only step **one large step** with a pivot foot to get the place the ball is passed. A caught pass is a point. Players work to get as many points as they can in a declared amount of time, for example you can put three minutes on the clock and see how many points partners can earn. Partners switch on the coach's call. Partner teamwork will be most effective with lots of enthusiasm and good tosses!

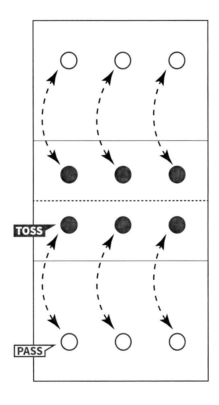

Cues

– Caught pass: 1 point
– Tosser can only take one step
Communicate:
– Tosser: "It's up," "I go! I go!"
– Passer: "My ball!"

REC+ Factor: 10 Team ups and then players switch

Pretzel
Passing Drill

Number of Players: Groups of Four   **Player Positions:** Group on Each Side of Net

Instructions

This drill has players in groups of four. There's a tosser with their back on the net and three passers about 15 feet out in front of the tosser. Like the look of a "Pretzel," players pass and switch with the player immediately next to them. The tosser switches up who they toss to. Passers stay **low** and open up to the other passers saying, "Go, go, go!" if it's not their ball. The player passing should always **claim** the ball, calling, "My ball, my ball, my ball!" If the ball is tossed to the middle passer, outside players must hold for a split-second as the middle passer picks who they will switch with. The pretzel-like movement continues until the coach yells out, "New tosser." This control passing drill can be timed for 30-45 seconds as the coach insists on staying low that entire time period.

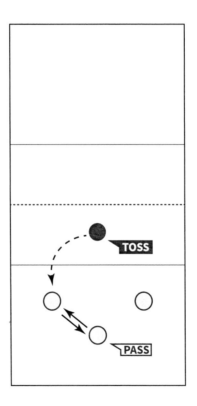

Cues

– Stay low
– Talk the entire time
– Celebrate at the end of each round
– After pass, passer switches with closest passer

Number of Players: All

Player Positions: Three Lines on Baseline

Instructions

From the three lines on the baseline, the first three players hustle out to the net and put their backs on the net. These players are targets. This coach toss drill will have players digging up to their target. Players dig and rotate up to the target spot. The initial targets turn and shag before returning to the digging lines. The coach can vary their degree of difficulty with the toss. Adding a score component to the drill will add a competitive twist, for example, 10 perfect digs to target. Remind your players to talk by claiming the dig and the up call at the time of the dig and remind your targets to call out, "I go! I go!" to catch the pass.

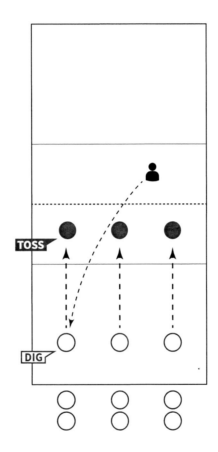

Cues

– Target gets one step
– All talk!
– Feet, feet, freeze
– "My ball!"

S5 Target Sets
Setting Drill

Number of Players: All   **Player Positions:** 5 Setting Positions Below

Instructions

In this drill **all** players are setters. Players are positioned in the drill with three setters in the back row and two setters in the front row. The coach tosses or free balls to the back row setters. The three back row setters (S1, S2, S3) set to S4, who is positioned in the setter's zone. S4 sets to S5, who is positioned in the Outside Hitter position and they shoot set the volleyball over the net. All setters work hard to get the ball up to the setter's zone. Solid footwork is important and the emphasis on **holding the follow-through** will result in better setting.

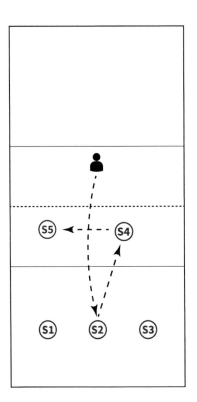

Cues

– S1, S2, S3 all set S4 who sets S5

Footwork:
– Jab and plant
– To net
– Net to left
– Pivot and square

Number of Players: All

Player Positions: Three Lines on Baseline

Instructions

Six hitters are placed on the floor and the coach tosses quickly to all six hitters. When a hitter successfully completes a hit the **team** earns one point. The team needs 10 points to win the drill. Players, during a bonus round minute, can earn two points if they meet the coach's call, for example: cut shot, cross court, off-speed roll shot. Players rotate by washing the drill. The coach can also assign a setter to come forward and receive a coach toss from behind the drill.

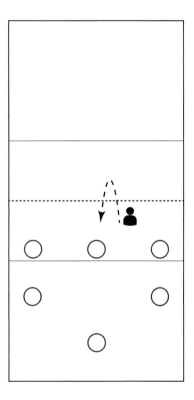

Cues

– Hit in: 1 point
– Bonus round: 2 points
– Footwork cues
– Alligator jumps

REC+ Factor: Bonus round and setter coming from back row

Jump Training x6
Hitting Drill

Number of Players: Partners

Player Positions: Six Stations Scattered

Instructions

The coach uses six station cards, file folders cut down and set up on edge or taped to cones, to identify six jump training exercises. The players are expected to work hard for the 30-45 seconds then jog between stations, clapping and demonstrating enthusiasm! The coach may demonstrate how hard work looks and what is expected for that short bout of time per each station.

The six stations are:

1) Front to back and side to side jumps

2) Three step hitting approach

3) Lateral slides or lunges

4) Jump rope for speed

5) 1-2 blocking footwork : baby step, cross-over step, sit, and jump

6) 12' agility drill or some type of direction-changing challenge

---

Number of Players: All   **Player Positions:** Six Players with Added Set

Instructions

This drill is designed to help the setter identify when they just can't get to a **bad pass**. The coach tosses a toss that is difficult or impossible for the setter to get to and the setter says, "Help! Help! Help!" The alternative setter does their best to put the volleyball out in front of a hitter. Hitters must communicate and work to successfully get the third hit over. This drill reminds players that **all players** need to be ready to set. The coach can rotate players around the floor or wash the drill, making sure all players start in the setting position. The coach reminds players to run with their hands free and to draw their setter's hands once feet are frozen.

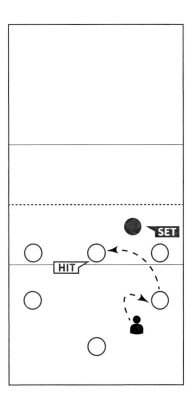

Cues

– Coach tosses bad pass
– May use three front row hitters or seven players
– "Head to ball"
– "Freeze and draw"

3 LoBL Combo Touches
Ball Control Drill

Number of Players: All   **Player Positions:** Three Lines on Baseline

Instructions

3LoBL formation will have the first three athletes stepping into the floor. The coach communicates a series of touches or skill sets desired, for example: free ball, dig, track and smack. Players then, as a team demonstrate those skill sets in the order the coach called out. A combination of skills will determine how the coach will toss. Players are expected to call out the skill to communicate back to the coach the skill set they should be doing. Coach can emphasize some general cues throughout the drill like, frozen-feet, snap to draw setter's hands, shoulder to the ball when hitting.

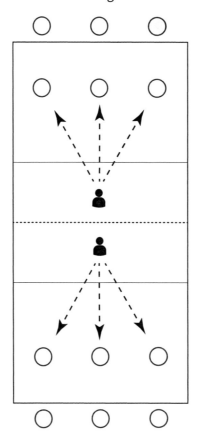

Cues

- Hip to the ball
- Fast toss
- Player call out their skill
- "Frozen feet" always priority

Coaches Commands:

- Pass
- Set
- Free ball
- Track and Smack

Number of Players: All

Player Positions: Baseline

Instructions

All players are on one baseline, ready to serve. With chairs set up to symbolize players, hula hoops or cones are placed in the spaces between the chairs. Players serve aiming for cones while avoiding the chairs, teaching the lesson that we want opponents to **move** to get to a serve. We don't serve to players, we serve to spaces between players. An emphasis should be placed on the solid serving routine.

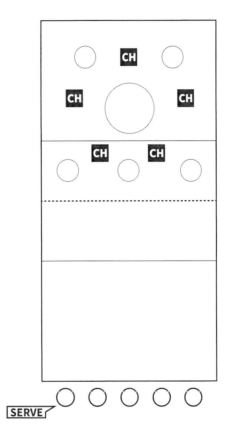

Cues

– Chairs: players
– Cones: space between players
– Don't serve chairs, serve cones
– Routine and rhythm

Serve Receive Rotations
Serve Receive Lesson

Number of Players: All

Player Positions: Six on Floor

Instructions

Players go from basic to serve receive without the volleyball, learning how to slide over, down, up to get in position for **serve reception**. The coach can begin the drill from three lines on the baseline and wash the drill or by simply placing players on the floor. Rotate around the floor so that all players experience each rotation and position. Coach says, "Basic!" (three back row, three front row) and "Serve Receive!" (serve receive formation).

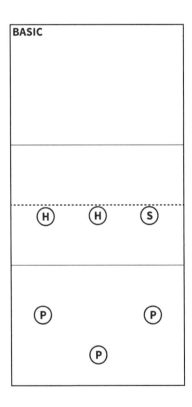
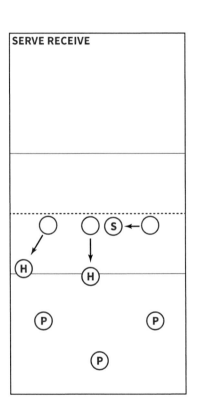

Cues

– Present each rotation
– Basic to "serve receive"

Number of Players: Groups of Three or Four

Player Positions: Serving Baselines

Instructions

The coach divides the team in either two or four teams. Ideally, this game is played on two courts but it can easily be played on one. When the game begins the teams are making as many serves over, 1 point per made serve, to 10 points. After 10 points, the serving team moves to the first open baseline. Once 10 more team serves are served, the team runs to the next service area. Making 10 team serves from four different baselines gets you to 40 serves and 40 wins the game! If you are only playing on one court - teams can serve five from both ends twice, totaling a game of 20.

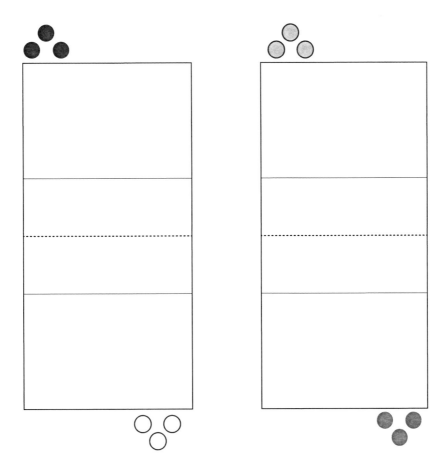

Cues

- Team moves as a unit to each baseline after 10 team serves
- The team who gets 10 from each baseline, or 40, wins
- Serve fast but focus on routine

Serve and Sprint
Serving Drill

Number of Players: Individual   **Player Positions:** Baseline

Instructions

Divide the team in half with each half on the serving baselines. Learning to "gain composure" after exertion, players serve and sprint to the opposite serving line. They reset their feet, take a deep breath, and start their routine. Once the player serves they practice calming down and being an effective server. The coach may put a certain amount of time on this challenge.

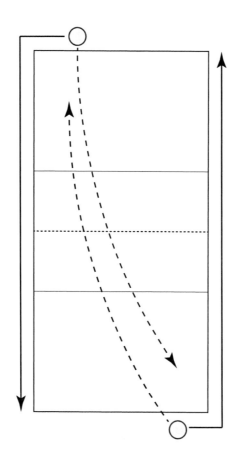

Cues

– Server's composure
– Exaggerate a deep breath to relax before serving

REC+ Factor: Conditioning drill, followed by composure

Number of Players: Partners

Player Positions: Both on Net

Instructions

Players have a partner. Both players start with their backs on the net. On the ball slap, the passing partner turns and back pedals to receive the toss from their partner. The first toss is short, just behind the 10' line. Once the first pass is completed, the passer back pedals to the longer distance on the baseline. Passers work to shuffle low and athletic and hop and freeze to pass the ball.

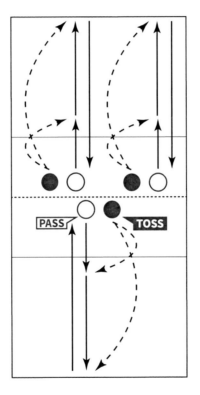

Cues

– One partner moves while the other tosses
– Two tosses: One short and one long
– Feet, feet, freeze
– Short: "Drop and pass"
– Long: "Shovel"

REC+ Factor: Passers learn to drop, cross, and hop-hop to get their feet set and frozen to deliver the pass

Touch Two
Defensive Drill

Number of Players: All   **Player Positions:** Two Lines on Baseline

Instructions

Players are organized in two digging lines. Two quick down balls or relatively hard throws are targeted at the digger. The digger digs two, shags, and returns to the digging lines. The coach emphasizes "low hands" and an aggressive desire to not let anything hit the floor!

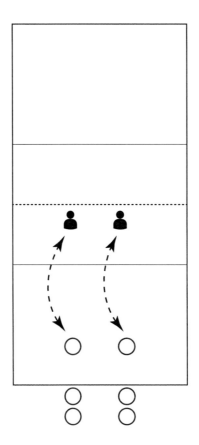

Cues

- "Step and stick"
- "Low hands"
- "Low Platform"
- "Hips above the ball"

         www.theartofcoachingvolleyball.com

Shuffle, Shuffle, Freeze "Dance"
Passing Drill

Number of Players: All

Player Positions: Evenly Spaced

Instructions

Players are positioned in a group formation in lines, with plenty of room. Like a team dance, players follow the coaches lead and call out the footwork. Players move together in a rhythm going six to eight different directions. The coach can define the directions prior to beginning. Players must stay low and get through the six to eight spots and recover back to the middle each time. Remember coaches to face the net or have your back to the players so they can truly mirror your moves.

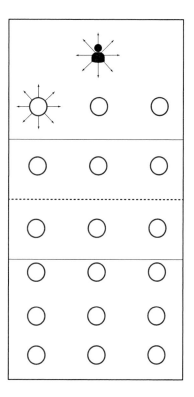

Cues

– "Dance" starts in ready stance on whistle
– Coach points the pattern and leads players in saying, "Feet, feet, freeze!" or "1, 2, freeze!"

REC+ Factor: Add a simulated movement of passing or setting at the completion of each footwork pattern.

Butterfly
Team Drill

Number of Players: Groups of Five to Seven

Player Positions: Across the Net

Instructions

This drill has five to seven positions filled on half the floor that create a "modified" butterfly drill. When done on both halves, it takes the look of butterfly wings. The coach or tosser (T) is positioned 5-15 feet behind the 10' line. They toss to the setter (S). The setter can self-set a couple of times to gain control or a more advanced setter can simply set out to the outside hitter (H). The hitter hits as the blocker (B) goes up to block and the digger (D) is deeper in defense working to dig or get the touch. Hitters are encouraged to hit at the digger. The digger can either turn and shag that ball, or the coach can add a shagger to go get that ball, while all other players rotate up a position. Players must learn to follow the pattern of the ball to know where to rotate. With the drill occupying both sides of the floor it does best when it is set up opposite or facing one another - again, forming that butterfly appearance.

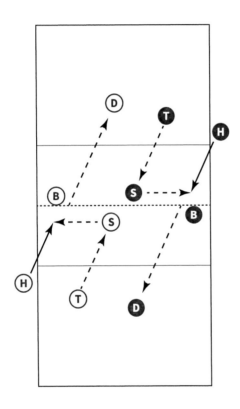 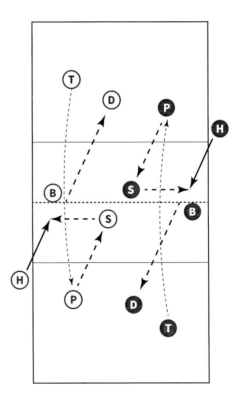

Cues

– Communicate
– Anticipate
– Alignment
– Feet first
– Tosser to Setter to Hitter to Blocker to Digger (to Shagger) to Tosser
– Tosser to Passer to Setter to Hitter to Blocker to Digger (to Shagger) to Tosser

Number of Players: All

Player Positions: 4 vs 4 wash

Instructions

The coach arranges players 4 vs 4 or in 4 lines on the baseline. The two teams compete to earn 10 points the fastest and win the round. A dig is worth 2 points, a kill is worth 1 point, a missed hit is minus a point, and if a ball hits the floor, also minus a point. Play on game until a team wins and then switch roles.

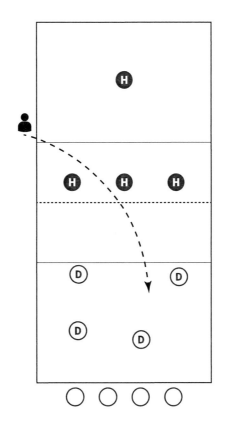

Cues

– First team to 10 wins
– "Anticipate and freeze"

Points:

– Dig: +2
– Ball hits the floor: -1
– Kill: +1
– Missed Hit: -1

Wall Work Series
Ball Control Drill

Number of Players: All

Player Positions: On Wall

Instructions

Wall work is for individual player development. Players find an area on the wall and move through a series of skills including: wall sets, wall down balls from a knee, wall down balls from standing, serving wall pins, serving wall deliveries or steady serving tosses, wall passing, and full wall serves , stepping off the wall 15-20 feet. This series can range from 30 seconds to 2 minutes per skill set.

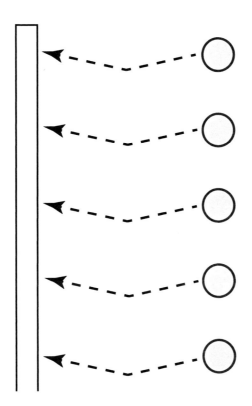

Drills

- Sets
- Down balls from knee
- Down balls standing
- Pins
- Tosses, shoulder on line
- Passes
- Serves

Number of Players: Groups of Three or Four

Player Positions: Three or Four Lines on Baseline

Instructions

Lines on the baseline will organize players for either 3 vs 3 play or 4 vs 4 play. Every touch is a point. The coach puts the ball in play with a free ball and players earn up to 3 points on one side, but the ball could be returned for additional points. Players play the free ball toss until it's defined dead and the players wash. The free ball toss always goes to side A. Players keep the **same teammates**.

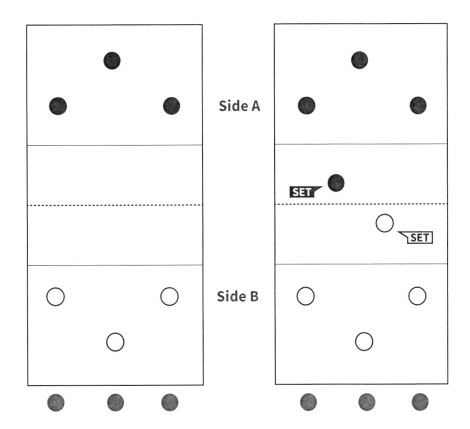

Cues

– 4 vs 4 wash
– Every touch is a point
– A touch is any contact with effort

REC+ Factor: a true three hits play where the hit goes over the net can result in a bonus 2 points, so the team would get 5 points instead of 3. The winning team does three push-ups while the non-winning team does 5 push-ups. The coach can reshuffle players and play another round!

Jump Train
Blocking Lesson

Number of Players: Partners

Player Positions: Partners at a Station

Instructions

These eight jump training stations are quite the workout! Have partners work hard at these eight stations.

The eight stations are:

1) Plyo step-close

2) 12' agility drill (pg.112)

3) Jump rope

4) 1-2 middle blocker footwork

5) One-step candy cane jumps (blocker candy canes hands up and over the net - straight up and back down)

6) Agility ladder work

7) One leg bounding (long skipping - skipping for height not length)

8) Two foot explosive ups.

Players should stay in the station for 30 seconds minimum and focus on good technique and speed reps. Players are expected to be enthusiastic and support one another between stations. Remind players to rotate with a jog and to never walk!

Number of Players: All

Player Positions: Scattered

Instructions

Players are divided up into four equal groups at four stations:

1) Vertical jump testing

2) Mini-hurdles

3) Agility ladders

4) 12' agility challenge

Players work hard for two to three minutes to work on their explosiveness, low movements, athletic stance, and always striving for sound jumper's feet! Coach emphasizes the importance of changing directions quickly when training and when playing the game!

Cues

– Powerful
– Explosive
– Low
– Changing directions fast
– Good jumpers

Four Corners
Passing Drill

Number of Players: All   **Player Positions:** Four Lines in Box Formation

Instructions

Players are equally divided into four groups and put in lines in a box formation. Players remember cross, line, cross, line. From a toss, the ball travels across to the diagonal line and that line passes back across to the "line" line. The coach can have the players go to the end of their line or follow their pass and go to the end of that line. Follow the illustration to see the details of how the drill flows. The coach emphasizes talking, moving, and being ready when in line since the drill moves quickly!

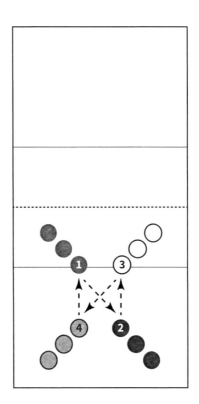

Cues

– Ball pattern: cross, line, cross, line
– Players start in four lines
– Feet, feet, freeze
– Draw "setter's hands" or stick your platform

Number of Players: All   **Player Positions:** 6 vs 6 Formation

Instructions

The transition fluidity drill is a walk-through type of drill that calls for players to use their imagination. Players will have specific places to rotate or move to as the coaches (two coaches needed) explain offense to hitter coverage to defense. The players are expected to repeat the transition they are in three times. Players say, "ready-ready" or "feet-feet" as they adjust to receive an imaginary free ball or "cover-cover" as they circle in to cover the hitter, or "down-down-down" to adjust and prepare on defense. The coach carries the ball around, lifting it and showing what situation is happening. Move in slow motion around the floor teaching the basic adjustments in transitioning. The coaches may begin tossing the ball to add a little speed and game-like movement to the transitions, but they players will only catch the volleyballs. Remember, players are expected to talk and communicate with every transition. The drill should look fluid-like in time.

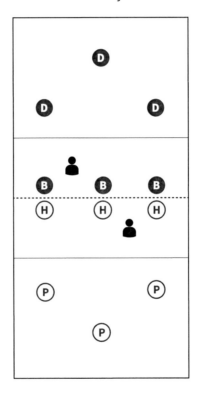

Cues

Players call out:
- Defense: "Down, down, down!"
- Coverage:" Cover, cover!"
- Offense: "Feet, feet!"

Three Deep
Serving Drill

Number of Players: All   **Player Positions:** Baseline

Instructions

Players serve as a **team**! All players are positioned on one baseline. Servers serve deep. The team is trying to get three deep serves **in-a-row**. Once this first serve lands in either zone 1, 6, or 5, two more must land deep to win the drill.

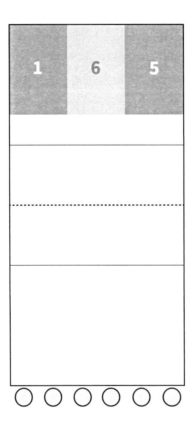

Cues

– Routine
– Rhythm
– "Punch"
– "Fast arm"

REC+ Factor: A serve that strikes any sideline is worth two deep serves in-a-row

---

Number of Players: All

Player Positions: Six Players On

Instructions

The coach assigns an outside hitter and five other players to cover the hit. The set can come from a coach's toss or the setter, if she's skilled enough. The coach holds up a "block," a football blocking pad works well, and the hit comes down off the block. Players dig the ball out of hitter coverage and play it out! Players are encouraged to talk: "cover-cover" "down-down-down" and remember to transition quickly to defense!

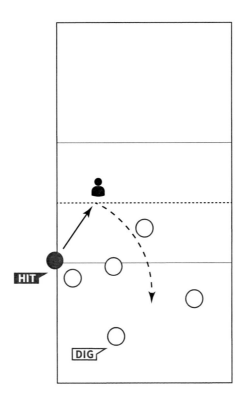

Cues

– Communication
– "Cover! Cover"

REC+ Factor: The coach can swing and hit into the blocking wall for more consistent digging touches.

Four Player Pass and Switch
Passing, Setting Drill

Number of Players: Groups of Four

Player Positions: Net to Baseline x2

Instructions

Players are put in groups of four in a box formation, with players facing one another. One player starts the drill by tossing directly across, not diagonal, and after the toss the partners next to one another switch. The ball always travels on the same path. The player receiving the toss passes back across to where the toss came from. Players essentially pass to the partner across from them and switch with he one beside them. Players are reminded to talk; "My ball, my ball," "Switch, switch, switch!" Players stay low and active and put the ball immediately back in play when the ball is dead.

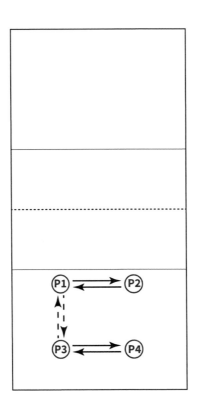

Cues

– Ball stays on the same path
– Talk fast
– "It's up!"
– "My ball!"
– "Go, go, go!"
– Switch, switch!"

Hitting, Defensive Drill

Number of Players: All

Player Positions: Hitting Lines

Instructions

The game Jail Break typically has all players serving but in this version, players are hitting off the coach's toss. Players that successfully hit the ball over the net return to the back of the hitting line and keep hitting, but a player who misses their hit must go to jail. In jail, hitters become diggers. To get out of jail and back into the hitting line, a player claims and digs the volleyball. The player whose ball was dug switches with the digger and goes to jail. The way to win the game is to be the last hitter swinging and get a kill against all teammates trying to dig you.

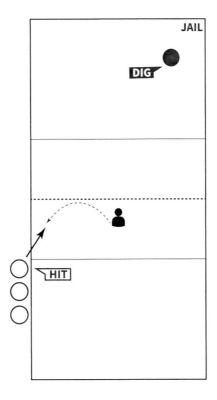

Cues

– All players hit outside
– **Good hit:** keep hitting
– **Miss:** off to jail
– **Ticket out of jail:** dig a hit ball
– **Hit is caught:** off to jail

REC+ Factor: the coach yells out "Jail Break" emptying out the jail and freeing all hitters

Free Ball 1,2,3
Passing Drill

Number of Players: All

Player Positions: Three Lines on Baseline

Instructions

As three players at a time enter the floor, the coach tosses a **second hit** and the team of three works hard to send an aggressive free ball over. Players pivot and turn a shoulder perpendicular to the net and aggressively send a **high and deep** free ball! Players send over a free ball and then shag or return to the lines. Players in line replace one another as passers abandon their position.

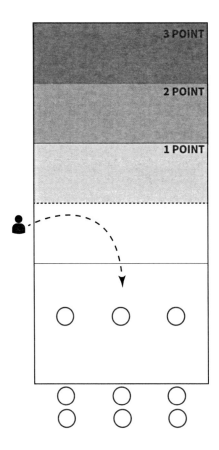

Cues

– Players pivot to free ball position to send over third hit
– High and deep is key

REC+ Factor: A points system divides the floor to emphasize the highest number of points to be awarded to the deepest free balls. Then make a team challenge of 20 points.

Serve One, Pass One
Serving, Passing Drill

Number of Players: All

Player Positions: One Line or Two Lines

Instructions

This combo-drill allows for quick body positioning and game-like switching of skills. Players are in two lines facing the coach, who will toss from over the net. Players all have a ball in their hand. When it's the next player's turn, that player will serve, then immediately step in to pass. Players should step into the floor quickly, widening their stance with each step. Hips then drop, drop, drop and hands do as well, preparing to pass. Players shag their **two** volleyballs, the serve and the pass, returning one to the cart and keeping the other for their next serve.

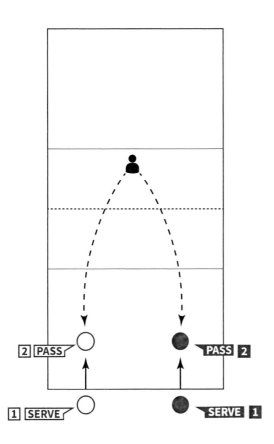
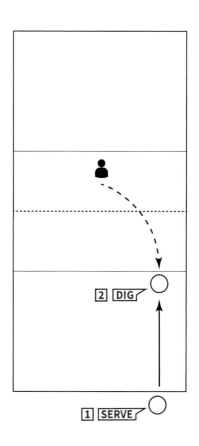

Cues

– Hustle onto the floor
– Get lower with each step
– Players can also dig the ball after their serve, as shown on the court above

Three in-a-row
Team Drill

Number of Players: All   **Player Positions:** Three Lines on Baseline

Instructions

This drill is organized with three lines on the baseline, bringing players out three at a time with the challenge of repeating the same skill three times in-a-row. For example three sets with the third set going over, three passes with the third pass going over. The goal is to get the three contacts in-a-row. Three digs in-a-row would wash the drill and get three more players on the floor.

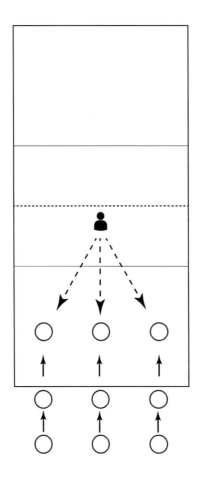

Cues

– Three in-a-row to wash
– Team goal is to get three different challenges
– Communicate
– Repeat coach's call

Number of Players: Groups of Five to Seven   **Player Positions:** Across the Net

Instructions

This drill has five to seven positions filled on half the floor that create a "modified" butterfly drill. When done on both halves, it takes the look of butterfly wings. The coach or tosser (T) is positioned 5-15 feet behind the 10' line. They toss to the setter (S). The setter can self-set a couple of times to gain control or a more advanced setter can simply set out to the outside hitter (H). The hitter hits as the blocker (B) goes up to block and the digger (D) is deeper in defense working to dig or get the touch. Hitters are encouraged to hit at the digger. The digger can either turn and shag that ball, or the coach can add a shagger to go get that ball, while all other players rotate up a position. Players must learn to follow the pattern of the ball to know where to rotate. With the drill occupying both sides of the floor it does best when it is set up opposite or facing one another - again, forming that butterfly appearance.

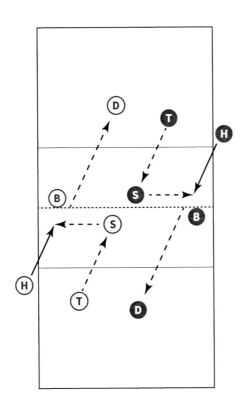 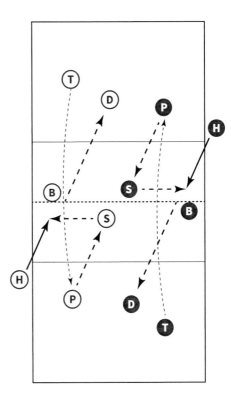

Cues

- Communicate
- Anticipate
- Alignment
- Feet first
- Tosser to Setter to Hitter to Blocker to Digger (to Shagger) to Tosser
- Tosser to Passer to Setter to Hitter to Blocker to Digger (to Shagger) to Tosser

Year 6

Save to Play
Team Drill

Number of Players: All

Player Positions: Three Lines on Baseline

Instructions

The coach puts the team in a 6 vs 6 formation and stands behind one baseline. The coach sends up a crazy toss! Players communicate to save the "bad pass" from the coach and **play it out**! Players on the other side of the net, in defense, are down and ready to dig and 6 vs 6 plays out to a dead ball. Players receive three "crazy first passes" from the coach and the drill washes. The coach places emphasis on transition volleyball and non-stop talking!

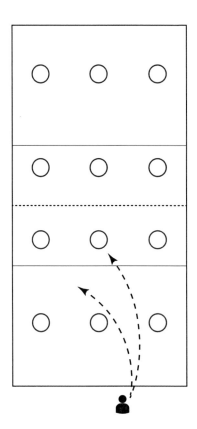

Cues

– Coach's toss is first contact
– Play the ball out
– After three tosses from coach, wash!
– Active feet
– Communicate
– Finish!

Number of Players: Partners

Player Positions: Across the Net

Instructions

Players are partnered up and across the net from one another, 10' line to 10' line. Players serve with great focus and body mechanics. After every five serves each or 10 total, players both have a ball to complete 10 "delivery" tosses each or 20 total. Players repeat the task: serve 10, deliver 20.

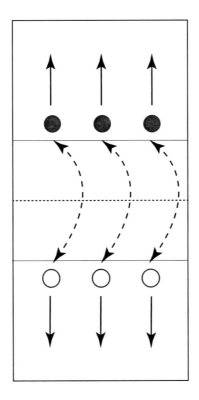

Cues

– Each player serves five and delivers 10
– Flawless controlled form
– No "Jumbo Shrimp Tosses"

Worksheets

Worksheets

Sticker Chart

The Sticker Chart is a fun way to get players engaged and reward their efforts. Each player gets a chart and puts their name on it. You then set your expectations for each skill for players to receive a sticker. For example, coach says, "50 popcorns and you've earned your sticker."

Popcorn: Players are given a certain combination of forearm popcorn, self-sets, floor down balls, passing or catching low, and top spins.

Sand and Punch: Players are underhand serving and "sand off" the striking area of their hand by sliding their thumb over and making a fist so that there is a solid contact area to serve the ball. Players then "punch" the ball.

Ready Position: Players are asked to get into their "ready position" with a wide base, feet ready to move, arms out and long, shoulders in front of toes. You can have them strike the ready position pose a certain number of times to earn their sticker.

Feet, Feet, Freeze: Players run or do jumping jacks and then "freeze" in the ready position. Try and get players to move their feet in this one to work on moving and then getting stopped to pass.

Track and Smack: Players toss super high to themselves and let the ball bounce once before smacking it over the net or into a wall with topspin.

Wrist Snaps: Players hit down balls into the floor.

Trophy Top: Much like Feet, Feet, Freeze, players can go from jumping jacks to "Trophy Top," demonstrating elbows above their ears to earn their sticker.

Serve Routine: Players work on the wall to individually to go through each step of the serve: two dribbles, step back, cool spin, one-two-punch.

Personal Best Score Card

The Personal Best handout is to help players understand setting goals and learning to complete with themselves. Players keep their results to themselves by keeping their papers face down. Coach challenges players with timed activities and players record their personal best.

1-3: Challenges timed for 30 seconds

4-6: Challenges timed for 40 seconds

Volleyball 10,000™

Volleyball 10,000™ is an incentive-based program that encourages daily touches based on the magic number 10,000 and the message that 10,000 hours can make you an expert. Volleyball 10,000™ has 10, 11 with the bonus, volleyball ball handling and muscle-memory fundamental movement exercises that players complete in sets of 20. This integrity driven program honors a player's initials as their word of completing each task. Players submit the Volleyball 10,000™ forms to **coachemuptexas.com** and are awarded recognition on the Volleyball 10,000™ Wall of Fame and a t-shirt, with cost only for the price of the t-shirt and the postage to mail. Coaches may use Volleyball 10,000™ as means of homework or offer it in the off-season or summer camps.

How Many Challenge

The How Many Challenge is a handout for players to document their best "in-a-row" scores as the clock is running. Players start trying to complete a task, counting how many they accomplish "in-a-row" before the clock runs out. For example, if a player is working on the "Passes to Yourself" challenge, they begin passing to themselves until they shank, if they got to 5 and there is still time left on the clock, they can try and beat their number. This timed challenge encourages fast-paced touches and help builds that competitive spirit.

Notecard Tournament

The Notecard Tournament is quick and fun. Round-robin format has players recording their timed games of competition on a 3x5 notecard. Players are not recording wins, but recording total points scored in the amount of playing time, suggested 5 to 8 minute sets. The complete set of instructions are below.

Notecard Tournament

Number of Players:	Groups of 3-6
Player Positions:	One team on each side of either a full court or a "short court", a court with dimesions you want.
Need:	3x5 notecards, pencils, court, and a ball.
How It Works:	This is a round robin tournament, everyone plays everyone. Coach sets time of each game before picking teams. Teams pick a name to put on their team card. Teams playing each other "Rock, Paper, Scissors" for serve. Players play until end of the time period. Remind players to announce the score before each serve. Teams always meet at the net to shake hands after the game. Points are recorded on their team card. Players report points, not wins or losses.
Additional Play:	After all teams have played each other, the two teams with the top points play each other for 1st and 2nd place, the next two scores play for 3rd and 4th, etc.

_____'S VOLLEYBALL SKILLS

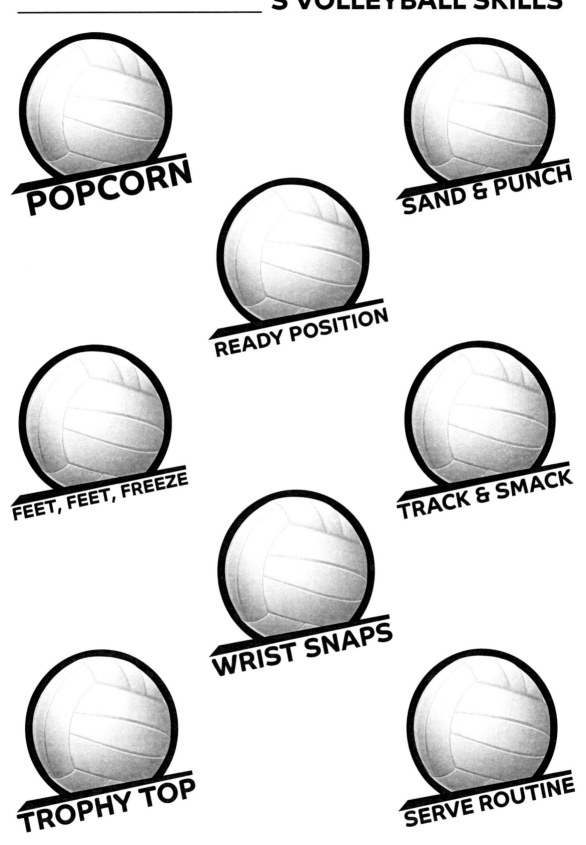

POPCORN

SAND & PUNCH

READY POSITION

FEET, FEET, FREEZE

TRACK & SMACK

WRIST SNAPS

TROPHY TOP

SERVE ROUTINE

Personal Best Score Card 1-3

_____'S PERSONAL BESTS

JUMPING

Jump Rope Rotations _____
_____
_____

Power Jumps _____
_____
Power Jumps _____

SKILLS

Floor Down Balls _____
_____
_____

Self Sets _____
_____

FUN

Knee ---- Knee _____
Pad ------- Pad _____
Slides ---- Slides _____

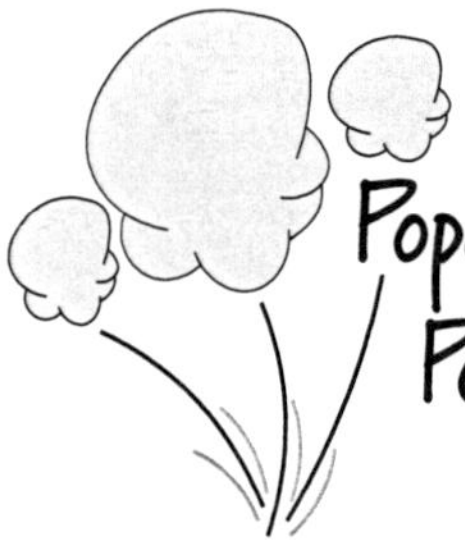

Popcorn Pops _____
_____

SPORTSMANSHIP

Teammate High 5 Five's _____
_____
_____

Pats On Backs _____
_____

_____'S PERSONAL BESTS

JUMPING

Speed Rope Rotations _____

_____

_____

One Foot Jumps

R:___ L:___
R:___ L:___
R:___ L:___

SKILLS

Wall Sets _____

_____

Wall Down Balls _____

_____

Floor Down Balls _____

_____

BALL HANDLING

Popcorn Pops _____

_____

_____

No-Mess Ups Challenge _____

_____

SPORTSMANSHIP

Teammate High Five's _____

_____

_____

Pats On Backs _____

_____

_____

Genuine Compliments
Nice!
Good job!
Great pass!
Keep it up!
Way to work hard!
That was a great hit!

_____

_____

_____

VOLLEYBALL 10,000™

PLAYER: _____ GRADE: _____

1. BALL SLAPS: NOT THUDS
      20____   20____   20____   20____   20____

2. POPCORN: ALTERNATING PLATFORMS
      20____   20____   20____   20____   20____

3. FLOOR DOWN BALLS
      20____   20____   20____   20____   20____

4. SERVING WALL PINS
      20____   20____   20____   20____   20____

5. SELF-SETS: SHAPING A PANEL ON AN IMAGINARY BALL
      20____   20____   20____   20____   20____

6. "4" SETTING DRILL
      20____   20____   20____   20____   20____

7. WALL SETS: WRIST WRINKLES AND FOREHEAD WINDOWS
      20____   20____   20____   20____   20____

8. SERVING ROUTINE
      20____   20____   20____   20____   20____

9. THREE STEP HITTING APPROACH: FOOTWORK TO SWING
      20____   20____   20____   20____   20____

10. BLOCK JUMPS: CANDY CANES WITH INVISIBLE BALL ELBOWS
      20____   20____   20____   20____   20____

BONUS : WALL SERVES
      20____   20____   20____   20____   20____

THE HOW MANY CHALLENGE

NAME: _____

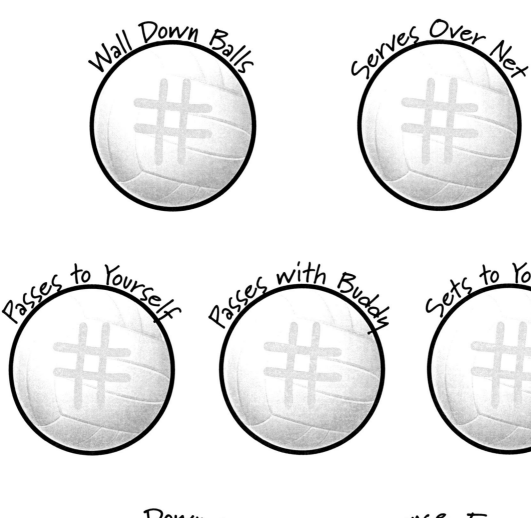

Wall Down Balls

Serves Over Net

Passes to Yourself

Passes with Buddy

Sets to Yourself

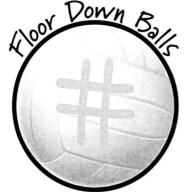

Floor Down Balls

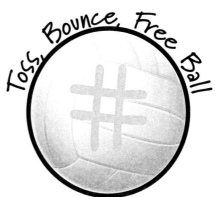

Toss, Bounce, Free Ball

Lessons

Quick Lessons

Free Ball	The players need to learn the body positioning for a free ball. Players will want to swing their platform to get the ball to go far but instead teach them to turn their bodies and drop the shoulder closest to the net to send the ball over high and deep.
Knee Pad Slides	Players run and slide on their knee pads. Players slide for distance. A toss can be added to encourage players to slide.
Lateral Footwork	Players shuffle while keeping the distance between their feet. Make sure players are not simply sliding and letting their ankles touch in the middle. Next players shuffle and then hop into or freeze in their ready stance.
Overhand Hitting	Players start with their non-dominant or opposite foot forward and their dominant or hitting hand big. Players move their feet to line their hitting shoulder up on the ball. While stepping with their opposite foot, players reach high making sure their elbow leads and making contact with their open hand on the ball. Players then "dry their fingernails" by snapping their wrists so that their middle finger points down to the floor.
Overhand Serving	Players start with 10 toes to the target, two dribbles, then step back with the same foot as their dominant hand, cool spin, ball in front of the hitting shoulder, hitting hand pulls back with four fingertips to the ceiling, then toss, step, punch. Players step with their opposite foot to get more power.
Passing	Emphasize players being low and in their ready stance with their hands always starting apart and coming together before they contact the ball.
Passing Form	Players pass with a wide base, feet outside their shoulders with their knees inside their feet. Players have their toes slightly turned in and are low as if they are sitting in a chair. Players have their platform out and relaxed with palms up and fingertips down. As the ball comes to the player, they put their hands together using either of the passing hands below.
Passing Hands	**Pancakes:** have players stack one hand on top of the other making sure they are flat and then have them roll their thumbs on top of the pancake stack. **Hot Dog:** have players make a fist with one hand and then have them wrap their other hand around the fist making sure their thumbs are flat on top.
Platform Austin Bat Thumbs	The Austin Bats are formed when the back of the thumbs are together. Players can open their hands and make a bat movement while keeping the back of their thumbs together.
Platform Strike Zone	Show players the sweet spot or strike zone of their platform, the section of their forearm between their wrists and elbows.

Practice Management	One Whistle: 10 toes, two eyes, with the ball on the floor. Two Whistles: huddle up, sit down, and hold onto your ball.
Ready Stance	Players have a wide base with their weight off their heels so that they are ready to move. Players should have their arms out and long with their shoulders in front of their toes. Players hands should be open with their palms slightly turned up with eight fingertips rolled down to the floor.
Self-Bumps	Self-bumps start with a players toss to themselves and then they begin passing to themselves. This requires the players platform angle to be up and down and not forwards.
Serve Punching	With a strong fist and with the players thumb off to the side, players pop the ball up off a bounce or their own toss.
Serve Receive	Go through the two formations described in the In-a-Nutshell Offense Drill on pg. 148. Walk through "pushing the setter up" and moving from basic defense to serve receive.
Setting	Coach demonstrates: **Setter's Feet:** feet shoulder width apart, knees slightly bent, and the right foot slightly in front **Setter's Hands:** hands shaping a panel of a volleyball and the player looking out from the top of their eyes through their setting window. **Setter's Finish:** follow through with two hands on a glass wall and not puppy paws with wrists snapped down or sea turtles with wrists and arms out.
Sprawling	Players start with a wider then normal base and let their hands find the floor first and then extend and lengthen to the ball, belly down. After they sprawl, players work on pushing up off the ground as fast as possible back into their ready stance.
Tossing	Tosses are short of the tosser's partner or the target. Coach may place a spot 2-3 feet out in front of their partner to help show them where the toss is supposed to go. Show players how high the toss should be and use the cue word "tossing rainbows."
Underhand Serving	Players start with 10 toes to the target, two dribbles, then step back with the same foot as their dominant hand, cool spin, drip of sweat: ball is placed low so that a drip of sweat could fall on top of the ball, then one, two, punch. Players may step with their opposite foot if needing more power.

Quick Drills

Quick Drills

10-5-1 Challenge	Players learn to go from multiple, quick, skill-based challenges to a controlled serve. Following 10 self-bumps and 5 floor down balls, players gain composure before going through their serving routine and serving 1 ball. Depending on time, players can repeat the series.
Ball Slaps	The players slap the ball 10 times working hard to hit the ball with their whole hand. Players work on making a slapping sound and not a thud. Players dribble the ball with their non-dominant hand and down ball with their dominant hand.
Coach Toss: Catch and Bump	From a coach's toss, players watch the volleyball as it hits the floor and bounces. The challenge is for players to catch the volleyball after the bounce, low to the floor with their thumbs up and long and strong arms.
Free Net Time	When players walk into the gym, give them four or five things they can do with a partner or two: down balls, serving back and forth, passing circle, popcorn, or other ball handling exercises.
Jump Rope	Players go through a series of jumping warm-ups using the jump rope: speed jump, explosive jumps, one-foot, alternating, side to side jumps, front and back. Players should grasp the concept of not jumping super high, unless doing the explosive jumps, but trying to clear the rope while turning the rope fast.
Net Throws	Players throw various sized balls: nerf, tennis, etc, with a high elbow making sure to step with their non-dominant foot.
Noodle and Balloon Strikes	Using half a pool noodle, players keep a balloon in the air by reaching high and striking the balloon.
Over the Net Rainbows	Players toss back and forth from the 10' lines over the net, working on underhand tossing using two hands with thumbs up on each side of the ball.
Partner Passing	With one partner a few feet off the net and the other a few feet in front of the baseline, the partners begin passing the ball back and forth always staying low and moving their feet.
Partner Setting	Same as Partner Passing but now players are setting back and forth.
Partner Spot Tossing	Partners toss back and forth working to toss rainbows short of their partner. The partner wants to either catch the ball as it falls or self-bump with a long and strong platform.
Partner Tossing	For two minutes, partners work together to toss back and forth counting the number of successful catches.
Serving For Correction	Players serve while the coach walks around and identifies one thing for a player to correct. Use the Troubleshooting Manual to help identify corrections to make.

Serve Receive to Finish	Six players serve receive the ball from a coach's toss and then play it out from serve receive to hitter coverage to defense.
Serving the Setter and Sub	Players learn the importance of serving to a specific spot or to a specific player. Give the player a spot or zone to focus on serving.
Serving Wall Fun	Add hula hoops or colorful sheets of paper to the wall as targets. Players have fun trying to hit the designated spots. Coaches can add point values to specific targets.
Serving Wall Targets	Identify different objects around the gym as targets to serve towards. For example, serving to make a basket or serving to hit a sign on the wall.
Speed Serve	Players serve the ball as quickly as possible with no routine. Have players keep track of how many they make over in either a timed amount or a certain number of balls. This number can be their goal to beat next time.
Team Ball Slaps	The whole team works together to complete the Ball Slaps.
Team Serves	All players grab a ball and run to the back line. After completing their serving routine, players serve the ball over the net. Each player runs and gets their ball and stands on the other side of the court until the coach signals for another serve. Count number of serves that land in.
Tennis Ball Wall Throws	Players throw a tennis ball against a wall focusing on a high elbow with their opposite foot forward stepping toward the wall.
Wall Bumps	Players pass back and forth using the wall as their partner.
Wall Down Balls	Players compete to see who can get the most wall down balls in-a-row.
Wall Pins	Players are standing close to the wall in their hitting stance. Players toss the ball high and try to pin the ball between their hand and the wall. Their contact point should ne high and they should have a big open hand.
Wall Serving	Players complete their full serving routine and serve the ball towards the wall.
Wall Sets	Players set back and forth using the wall as their partner.
Wiggle TIme	Players have fun with their ball. Coach can choose between down balls, self-sets, wall work, etc.
Wind Sprints	Players run from the baseline to the 10' line on the same side of the court and then back to the baseline. Next, players run from the baseline to the net and back. Then, to the 10' line on the other side of the court and back to the baseline. Last, players run from the baseline to the opposite baseline and back.

Volleyball Glossary

Volleyball Glossary

Skill	Cues	Definition
Passing		
Body Alignment	Hips to the Ball	Getting middle of body to ball
Platform Hands	Hot Dog in a Bun	One hand is out with the thumb up and a fist Other hand wraps around first hand Put thumbs together and push to the floor
Platform	Long and Strong Be the Board	Lengthen or extend your platform Elbows locked and thumbs to the floor No swinging Keep distance between hands and hips
Platform Passing Shrug	Alligator View	Players shrug their shoulders around their jaw like an alligator rising out of the water
Ready Position	1-2-45-8	Relax 1" at knees 2" bend at waist 45° platform 8 fingertips to the floor, thumbs down
Passing Footwork	Feet, Feet, Freeze	1, 2, Step to get to every ball
Passer's Feet	Railroad Tracks	Parallel feet, shoulders over toes, hands apart
Contact	Extend and Lengthen	Footwork is stopped earlier than most think Distance yourself from the ball so at contact you have a long triangle base between your hands, shoulders, and hips
Follow Through	One Mississippi Hold	Players hold their platform for a one-Mississippi
Serving		
Routine	10 Toes to the Target Step Back, Cool Spin Pull and Pause Toss, Step, and Punch	Square up to the desired area Drag right foot back while you spin the ball Pull punching hand high off top of the ball Toss, step, and punch
Striking to Contact Form	Elbow Starts Up High Elbow by the Eye Thumb by the Thigh Palm to the Sky	After "pull," striking hand comes back, elbow leads Elbow comes out first Thumb follows through by the thigh Continued follow through puts palm to the sky
Float	Drop and Pop	Drop the elbow 1 inch, no follow through
Top Spin	Dry Your Fingernails	Focusing on "middle finger to the floor" High reach with frozen and exaggerated hold

Volleyball Glossary

Skill	Cues	Definition
Setting		
Hand to Setter's Window	Draw	Hands are quickly brought up, close to the body
Pre-Set Hand Placement	Setter's Window	Thumbs to eyebrows, see through the window
Receiving	Shape a Panel	Hands should shape the volleyball A panel is a group of 3 smaller horizontal pieces First fingers and thumbs should find corners
Full Extension	Load and Lengthen	Load the hips by dropping your center of gravity Extend from ankles to knuckles
To the Ball	Circle Belly Button Run and Draw	Hands should be at waist level Run normal with hands not above head
Follow Through	No Sea Turtles No Puppy Paws Only Mime Hands	Extend out not to the sides No finishing with wrists or hands down Hands are firm, fingers spread and both flat
Zone Positioning	To the Net and Left	Finding the setter's zone is a priority Players get to the net with their right shoulder Travel left to the ball
Hitting		
Ready Position	Runner's: To Your Mark, Get Set, Go	Hitter's weight forward, hips dropped, ready to run
Upper Body	Mr. Snuffleupagus 90˚ Elbows Raise the Roof Mountain Skier Trophy Top Track and Smack	Ready position arms are hanging like a trunk Ready to throw arms up Arms throw out Palms to the sky Arms snap to elbows above ears Off hand tracks ball and lines shoulder up to ball
Footwork	Weight Forward	Three step: Left, Right, Left (right-handed)
Adjustment Step	First Step to the Ball	Shoulder to the ball with ball out in front
Step, Close	Parallel Foot Brake	Left foot (right-handed) parallel with net
Wrist Snap	Middle Finger to Floor	Snap while reaching with a high elbow

Volleyball Glossary

Skill	Cues	Definition
Aggressive Free Ball		
Body Positioning	Shoulder's Perpendicular	Perpendicular to the net, turn and drop shoulder
Weight Transfer	Rocking Chair Legs	Rock back foot to front
Contact and Execution	High and Deep	Free balls should land in the back part of the court
Down ball and Free ball	Trophy Top and High Snap	Shoulder on the ball and middle finger to floor
Digging		
Body Alignment	Hips to the Ball	Get middle of body behind the ball when possible
Upper Body	Inside Shoulder Dropped	Long and strong platform, thumbs to floor
Footwork	Step and Stick	Step 45° towards ball and get long
Blocking		
Hands	Moose Antlers	Roll thumbs up, spread fingers, and shape ball
Hips	Drop and Sit	Bottom behind your heels
Feet	Best Jumper's Feet	Player find their best jumping feet
Jump	Candy Cane	Up and over the net, curve over
Footwork	Baby, Cross, Sit, Up	Baby: Small step to slightly open hips Cross: Long step in front Sit: Drop hips to jump Up: Candy cane over the net and antenna seal
"J" Release		
Footwork	Drop, Cross, Hop, Set	"J" move from basic defensive position to adjust Front row: Release blocker footwork Back row: Left and right back adjust to hitter
Transition Release	Blocker to Hitter	"J" move without the curl Drop, Cross, Hop, Set

Troubleshooting Manual

Troubleshooting Manual

Outcome or Error	Possibilities	Corrections
Serving		
Ball going into the net	Over striding on toss	Shorten stride to a step
	Toss too far in front	Shorten and relax tossing elbow
	Toss too low	Raise toss one inch
	Elbow too low	Raise elbow one inch
	Power from hips	Open and close faster
	Control of punch or contact	Drag back toe
Ball going deep or out of bounds	No wrist snap	Dry those fingernails
	Speedy arm	Control contact and slow arm
	Alignment	Fire cross court from corner
Passing		
Spin on the ball	Not frozen	Hold follow through
		No swinging through
Low trajectory	Incorrect platform angle	Shovel higher by raising platform
		Sit lower
	Weight too far on toes	Settle in prior to contact
High trajectory	Incorrect platform angle	Shovel lower by adjusting platform
		Platform below hips
		Fast knee extension
		Lower on contact
Ball not getting to net or target	Not enough legs	Faster and more accurate lift
		Deeper pre-contact position
	Not enough shrug	Get shoulders more involved
Ball shanking left or right	Uneven platform	Thumbs together
		Platform long and strong
	Alignment	Hips and shoulders to the ball
Ball going behind passer	Improper body positioning	Hips to the ball
	Platform flat or too high	Lower platform
	Not frozen	Feet set with a solid foundation
Setting		
Flat and splat sound	Receiving ball uneven	Level shaping hands
	Hands too close	Cover the ball
	Fingers too close	Shape a panel
	Ball not on finger pads	Too much palm or tips

www.theartofcoachingvolleyball.com

Outcome or Error	Possibilities	Corrections
Setting Continued		
Ball spinning	Follow through	Consistent, steady receive
		Hands exaggerate at extension
	Receiving too quickly	Allow ball to come into position
	Unsolid base or footwork	Get set and balanced under ball
	Uneven hands	Draw hands together and level
Not going out far enough	Extension is sluggish	Faster, sharp, intentional rise
	Trajectory	Extend at an ideal angle
	Receiving incorrectly	Setter's window
Ball in hands too long	Not enough wrist	More wall and speed work
		Optimize speedy extension
	Receiving too high or low	Placement is set and steady
Hitting		
Timing	There too soon or too late	Repetition and experimenting
	Behind the ball	Leave sooner and be explosive
	Early	Repetition with varying set heights
	Consistency for confidence	Controlled tossing to same spot
Ball into the net	Late arrival	Leave sooner
	Out on ball of feet	Weight more centered
	Jumping too far forward	Encourage more jump rope
	Strike is too low	Contact ball when it is above net
	Elbow or arm is low	More muscle memory off the net
	Miss hit	Ball not aligned on shoulder
Hitter in the net	Coming in on toes	Stronger step, close
	Swinging too much	Shorten follow through to wrist snap only
	Set position	Pull ball off net
Ball not going down	Wrist snap	Middle finger to the floor
Hit not aggressive	Hips and shoulders	Feet and base turned on step, close
		Ball in front of hitting shoulder
		Adjust plant step to be parallel
		More external oblique training
	No torque	Open and close chest and hips
		Throw shoulders closed faster

Troubleshooting Manual

Outcome or Error	Possibilities	Corrections
Digging		
Inconsistent contact or delivery	Alignment and Positioning	Firm, solid, and frozen platform Shoulders remain firm and solid
Ball shanking	Net shoulder No swinging Arms adjusted to angle	Drop inside or net shoulder Stick the platform and hold Level platform
Ball shooting to net	Platform trajectory	Drop hips and lower hands
Not getting to ball	Step and stick	Prioritize stepping to ball
Blocking		
Slow to the ball	Watching the ball	Identify set and go Seek hitter's shoulder Repetition of lateral movements Longer drop step
In the top of the net	Wristy	Hold form and have strong hands Candy cane up and over the net
In the net on the way up	Elbows spreading Dropping hands	Hold true to candy cane form Hands stay above ears and eyes
Ball dropping directly in front	Extending straight up	Extend up and over
Unbalanced block	Base or footwork not set	Sit before jumping Lower final step before you slow

Fundamental Skill Progressions

Fundamental Skill Progressions

Skills	1	2	3	4	5	6
Free Skill Time	x	x	x	x	x	x
Player Behavior and Expectations	x	x	x	x	x	x
General Footwork, Feet, Freeze, Shuffle	x	x	x	x	x	x
Muscle Memory Warm-up Throws			x	x	x	x
Ball Juggling Challenges	x	x	x	x	x	x
Floor Down Ball Work	x	x	x	x	x	x
Wall Work	x	x	x	x	x	x
Underhand Tossing	x	x	x	x	x	x
Communication Terms	x	x	x	x	x	x
Identifying when Receiving or Not Receiving	x	x	x	x	x	x
Calling or Claiming Responsibilities	x	x	x	x	x	x
Three Hits Objective and Drill Work			x	x	x	x
Underhand Serve	x	x	x	x	x	x
Overhand Throwing	x	x	x	x	x	x
Overhead Striking Challenges	x	x	x	x	x	x
Jumping and Striking	x	x	x	x	x	x
Overhand Serve				x	x	x
Under and Overhand Serving Routine			x	x	x	x
Place Serving				x	x	x
Jump Serving						x
Passing Hands and Platform	x	x	x	x	x	x
Passing Stance and Ready Position	x	x	x	x	x	x
Passing Form and Hip Alignment			x	x	x	x
Passing Basic Shuffle Footwork	x	x	x	x	x	x
Controlled Passing				x	x	x
Target Passing				x	x	x
Free Ball: first Hit	x	x	x	x		
Free Ball: 3rd Hit				x	x	x
Floor Contact Intro, Knee Pad Fun	x	x	x	x	x	x
The Volleyball Floor	x	x	x	x	x	x
Floor Rotations				x	x	x
Net Zones						x
Set Heights					x	x
Setter's Zone				x	x	x
Agility Challenges	x	x	x	x	x	x
Agility Assessments					x	x
Target "Stopping"	x	x	x	x	x	x
Running to Draw				x	x	x
Setting Intro	x	x	x	x	x	x
Setter's Hands			x	x	x	x
Setter's Window	x	x	x	x	x	x
Setter's Feet	x	x	x	x	x	x
Follow-through and Cover				x	x	x
Setting Height and Net Placement				x	x	x
Quicks, Slides, Back Row, Back Sets, Dumps						x

Skills	1	2	3	4	5	6
Overhead Tracking and Smacking	x	x	x	x	x	x
Trophy Top Striking Form	x	x	x	x	x	x
Down Ball Wall Work			x	x	x	x
Two Step Hitting Approach				x	x	x
Three Step Hitting Approach				x	x	x
Four Step Hitting Approach				x	x	x
Varying Hitting Speeds and Contacts	x	x	x	x	x	x
Hitting Angles					x	x
Target Hitting					x	x
Tips					x	x
Cut Shots						x
Passing and Digging Difference					x	x
Digging Stance				x	x	x
Step and Stick Digging Footwork				x	x	x
Digging Ups					x	x
Digging Placement						x
Sprawling					x	x
Rolling Basics						x
Jumping Rope	x	x	x	x	x	x
Jump Training				x	x	x
General Plyometrics						x
Dynamic Warm-up	x	x	x	x	x	x
Static Stretch	x	x	x	x	x	x
1, 2 Step Block Training				x	x	x
Three Step Block Jumping						x
Transition Defensive Blocking Intro					x	x
Transition Footwork					x	x
Solo vs Double Block Footwork						x
Transition Volleyball					x	x
4-2, 5-1, 6-2 General Info and Differences						x
Player Roles					x	x
Setter second Hits					x	x
Rotations						x
3 Hits: Offense to Hitter Coverage to Basic						x
Basic Middle Back Defense					x	x
Basic Rules: Officials, Lines, Judges Calls				x	x	x
Official Whistles and Calls				x	x	x
Time Outs and Huddle Behavior				x	x	x
Bench Behavior	x	x	x	x	x	x
Game Sportsmanship	x	x	x	x	x	x
Coin Flip and Captain's Role				x	x	x
Substitution Rules				x	x	x
League or Recreation vs Federation					x	x

Drill Index

Drill Index

Drill Index